LIVING THERAPY SERIES

Counselling Victims of Warfare

Person-Centred Dialogues

Richard Bryant-Jefferies

Radcliffe Publishing
Oxford • Seattle

Radcliffe Publishing Ltd
18 Marcham Road
Abingdon
Oxon OX14 1AA
United Kingdom

www.radcliffe-oxford.com
Electronic catalogue and worldwide online ordering facility.

_____

British Library Cataloguing in Publication Data

A catalogue record for this book is available from the British Library.

ISBN 1 85775 721 1

Typeset by Aarontype Ltd, Easton, Bristol
Printed and bound by TJ International Ltd, Padstow, Cornwall

Contents

Foreword

In the Armed Conflict Report of 2000 the peace group, Project Ploughshares, noted that there were 40 designated armed conflicts taking place in 36 countries. Sixteen in Africa, 14 in Asia, two in Europe, two in the Americas and six in the Middle East. In the conflict between Kashmir/India and Pakistan there were an estimated 65 000 deaths. In the Ethiopia/Eritrea conflict (at the time of writing violence has been rekindled in Ethiopia) estimates were that over 50 000 people have died. In other areas, such as Nigeria, violent conflict is ongoing (in the Northern territory), and there are regular violent flare-ups in the oil rich parts of the south. We know of the media coverage of violence in the Sudan, Zimbabwe, Ethiopia, and Iraq. We see little of the rest.

In the West we have a very different world — we think. We can choose not to watch the news ('too sad', 'too negative', 'too miserable'). We can cheer ourselves up with retail therapy when we feel a bit down. We can be rooted to the spot with shock when warfare is brought into our midst (the Twin Towers), or when troops sent out against our collective will (to Iraq) come back with stories and experiences that leave us without words to respond; or in Northern Ireland (with over 3250 deaths between 1969 and 1998) where we could pretend that it wasn't happening as long as it didn't affect the mainland.

We can perhaps pretend that wars in other countries have little to do with us, even though Britain sends troops as part of UN peacekeeping forces throughout the world.

In the West we are very good at pretending that everything is OK as long as we don't get too stressed (although therapists know of the extensive number of young people self harming, or who have experienced abuse, low self-esteem and significant distress). As a society, we can even try and ignore the problems in our own country.

In the therapy room I see children and teenagers, women and men, who have experienced beatings, abductions, rapes, torture, deliberate and violent attempts on their lives. They have witnessed the violent deaths of members of their families by sudden or the slowest means. Some of the young women bear children as a result. Some were forced as children to kill or be killed as child soldiers. Some young people talk about walking through their towns or villages stepping over the bodies of the dead. They have seen so many dead that sometimes they need to re-enact what they have seen.

Sometimes we sit together in silence, sometimes we sit and giggle at the things that make us all laugh. Sometimes it takes time for a session to end, as I try to gently bring this person or that back emotionally into the room; to look at me and know that we are here and not there.

For us as therapists we need to understand that the statutory services are not geared up to deliver a nationwide service to people in the UK who have experienced war first hand. We also need to be aware that many people escaping violence and fear are in the UK seeking asylum under the Human Rights Convention, and that if their claim fails, they may not be permitted to access the statutory services as a 'failed asylum seeker awaiting removal' (even though their case may be successful on appeal). Our UK policies may cause considerable emotional and psychological distress in addition to the traumas originally experienced.

How do we, then, work therapeutically with people whose experiences may be so different from our own, whose culture, country of origin, religion or philosophy may shape so many different frames of reference?

Richard refers to research which indicates that there is no specific 'best' therapeutic approach, but that it is the relationship between the therapist and the client which is helpful to the client. Therapeutic work with people who have been impacted by all that war is demands that the therapist is grounded, congruent and valuing of the client. How else could a therapist work with someone who has experienced violence from one faction or ethnic group (for example, the Hutus), and later in the day work equally as empathically with someone from that ethnic group (a Hutu) but who has experienced violence at the hands of someone from the ethnic group of the client you saw in the morning (a Tutsi)? How else could the therapist see a Kurdish young man in the morning and an Iraqi Arab in the afternoon whilst valuing and being open to them equally. The prizing and valuing of each and every client, extending empathy into each different frame of reference, whilst remaining congruent and accepting of the uniqueness of each individual, with a willingness to be open to see the world through their eyes, are the paramount requisites for this work.

Victims, or survivors, of wars (or 'hostilities', 'ethnic cleansing', 'inter-state disputes') experience considerable and ongoing trauma responses which are difficult to tolerate in the self and which threaten their sense of themselves as human beings. It is time to consider what is the best that we can offer to them.

Miriam Hollis
Founder and Director
The Sankofa Foundation
(a project for clients seeking asylum or who have refugee status)
Co-ordinator, Space2Be Counselling Service
June 2005

Foreword

It is a privilege for me to work with asylum seekers and refugees. Every time I listen to a new client I have overwhelming feelings of sadness and compassion, and I ask myself, 'How can one human being cause such suffering to another human being?'. These clients' feelings of hatred, anger and revenge can feel overwhelming to the listener. Yet as person-centred counsellors we learn how to listen in a non-judgemental way. It is not always easy but our training and level of self-awareness form the basis of our ability to do this sensitive and challenging work.

Counselling Victims of Warfare widens our understanding of how to apply the therapeutic values of the person-centred approach. It offers the reader scenarios which show clearly the reality for those who are affected by the atrocities and horrors of war. Whilst no counselling training or text book of interventions can ever fully prepare us, Richard shows us how we can deal with what can be a real struggle both as a supervisor supporting the counsellor, and as the counsellor walking beside her client in her painful journey to reconcile the bad, the evil and the goodness, and to find a sense of acceptance.

What Richard has written is essentially an affirmation of the potential value of the person-centred approach in working with clients who have suffered inhumane actions. In the first part, in which a victim of the war in Bosnia attends counselling, we see how the counsellor enables the client (Ania) to explore her inner world by focusing sensitively on Ania's feelings and responding to her readiness to engage in the therapeutic relationship. The healing process begins. The atrocities of war cause trauma, which creates chaos in people's lives, and this chaotic hurt leaves people speechless, voiceless, bewildered and silenced. The counselling enables Ania to make a coherent narrative out of painful events, so deeply buried that they completely disable her emotionally.

The author demonstrates the way that the person-centred approach can be used to support a traumatised client in telling her painful story, enabling her to describe her own suffering and empowering her to find the voice to communicate the way it was, and is, for her. Slowly she is able to reflect upon her life and how it can be now. The powerlessness and helplessness of her trauma have left their mark but we are able to follow her journey. This book illustrates how a person's spirit, the essence of their uniqueness and individuality are, when given the space, time and attention, able to re-awaken.

Counselling Victims of Warfare is a valuable tool to help prepare counsellors (and others) to work with clients who have experienced horrifying actions from another human being. A sense of horror can sadden and affect the counsellor. For the client, their intimate knowledge of what one human being can do to another, and what they can become a victim of, is revealed. It is difficult to comprehend how any fellow human being could behave in such a way.

There are no blue prints or right ways to do this work, but the application of the values and attitudes of the person-centred approach and methodology illustrated here can add to the counsellor's own knowledge, experiences and own self-awareness, and as we see in the text, play a vital role in enabling the client's voice to become her catalyst to heal and find herself again.

Menna Yarwood
Person-centred counsellor working with refugees and asylum seekers
North Sheffield Primary Care Trust
June 2005

Preface

When I attended a conference of the Association for the Development of the Person-Centred Approach in Manchester I met a person from America, Muhyiddin Shakoor, who had worked in Bosnia in the 1990s during the war. He ran a workshop at the conference and I think it will stay with me forever. He offered the participants different scenarios, each realities from working with people affected by the horrors of war. The scenarios were horrific, the kind that you do not meet on a daily basis in your counselling room at home or in a GP surgery, and certainly nothing that most training courses include as issues to deal with. The atmosphere in the room changed as we all tried to get our heads, and our hearts, around what we were reading.

We were asked how we would cope. There was silence in the room. It was Annie Thompson, another person-centred counsellor, who responded first, and in a way that certainly spoke for me, and probably captured what many other people were feeling in the room. 'I'd either be shit hot, or crap.' I was nodding, with tears in my eyes, not knowing either whether I would have been able to cope, or not.

The facilitator used the scenarios to illustrate how, when working with people at the really horrifying end of human experience, there are no techniques, no clever words to say, no textbook interventions to make. All that you can offer is yourself, another human-being, touched and affected by what you are hearing, unable to truly understand what the client has gone through, and is going through, but striving to convey some degree of appreciation of the depth of feeling that is present. And of course, to be open to your own thoughts and feelings, the experiencing within your own nature that is breaking into awareness as you seek to connect with the client's inner world. And, it goes without saying, to offer unconditional positive regard and warm appreciation for the person seeking to come to terms with their experiences.

As I embark on this book, I know that it is the one book that I do not want to write. I know that as I begin this narrative I will need to engage with images and feelings that should not be the experience of a human-being, but which, all too sadly, are commonplace in so many parts of the world. Part of me wants to deny the reality of the atrocities that are perpetrated by human-beings upon other human-beings and, I think it is reasonable to say, in particular by men upon women, though not exclusively so. But to do so is to deny a reality of human experience that must be acknowledged and to which I/we must open ourselves. Part of me wants to shrink back from writing it, and wants to say, 'there's another theme, there are lots of other topics, write them first. This one can wait'. The truth is, though, that it cannot. Too many people continue to be, and to become, victims of warfare, military and civilian, the victims of torture, of rape, the refugees, the bombed, the burned and the mutilated, and who carry with them emotional scars which can take so long to heal, if healing is truly possible or the right word to use.

It is not my intention in this book to shock, I do not want to overstep the mark and lose the reality. I want the reader to be touched, affected, but only so that through their reactions and experiences they may perhaps begin or extend their own process of personal development and enhance their capacity as a human-being to sit with other human-beings who have suffered extreme trauma.

In this book there is material to inform the training process of counsellors and others who seek to work with people experiencing this type of trauma. *Counselling Victims of Warfare: person-centred dialogues* is intended as much for experienced counsellors as it is for trainees, although working with clients who are victims of warfare is likely to require counsellors with some degree of experience. It provides real insight into what can occur during counselling sessions. I hope it will raise awareness of, and inform, person-centred practice within this context. Reflections on the therapeutic process and points for discussion are included to stimulate further thought and debate.

I do wish to point out that I have not focused so much on the refugee experience and the issues associated with asylum seeking. Whilst this area of work overlaps for so many victims of warfare, I have chosen to work with the traumatic impact on the client of their experiences, and the emotional and psychological effects. I am grateful to Miriam Hollis for sharing her experience with me of the plight of refugees and asylum seekers that she works with. She emphasised how for many clients there will be so much added complexity. Many victims of warfare are asylum seekers, war refugees seeking asylum from their experience. Yet they can find themselves faced with a harsh, authoritarian and bureaucratic system, their hopes for a better future undermined, and their self-esteem that is already low, at risk of descending further. To be brought to a country (perhaps at great expense) with hope in your heart of safety and a new start only to find yourself at risk of return, unable to understand the language and the culture, and knowing that return may mean death or torture and to then find yourself labelled as a problem in the media and for politicians, can only induce further fear and anxiety, exacerbating what is already present.

Added to this, asylum seekers can be dispersed to other towns without warning, regardless of whether they are in therapy/treatment. If their claim to asylum is refused their benefits are stopped and there is then little or no way to access healthcare. There can be fear of the authorities. For example, the raped and now pregnant refugee who is entitled to access healthcare may not see the midwife out of her fear of being reported and returned to a country where, in countries exercising Sharia law, she could be at risk of a death penalty.

There are on-going attempts for greater clarity so that doctors and midwives can be clear concerning their position for treating asylum seekers, or those whose asylum has been refused. So little can be offered, it seems, and there is so little training and experience within mainstream healthcare. Few health authorities have specialist support available for this group of people which results in not just the psychological but also the physical effects of their trauma going unrecognised and untreated. The need for translators, in particular, is desperate, together with appropriate emotional support for the translators themselves who become exposed to the traumatic horrors at least as much as the counsellor, yet without the training, personal development and supervision and support that the counsellor receives. The Medical Foundation for Survivors of Torture is dependent on voluntary counsellors and doctors. Person-centred working is not so clearly recognised in this area of work and yet the theoretical nature of the approach seems, on the face of it, to have so much to offer to therapeutically counteract what has been, and is being, experienced by the client.

Counselling Victims of Warfare: person-centred dialogues also addresses the impact of warfare on the military combatant. Coming to terms with experiences within the battlefield: stress, fear, loss of friends and comrades, guilt at having survived, as well as for some knowledge of the abuse of prisoners and of rape perpetrated, can be difficult. This can be particularly so where the person comes from a military family, or from a community where there is a strong association with the military; where they may have left as heroes and return feeling less than heroic, their self-concept now very much at odds with how others want to see them.

Counselling victims of warfare is a huge topic. This book explores some aspects in terms of person-centred theory and practice and has value to health and social care professionals who, whilst they may specialise in other areas, may be required at times to work with people who have been affected by warfare. Not everyone can be a counsellor or will wish to engage at depth at a human and emotional level with victims of warfare. I hope that this book addresses a range of themes and leaves you, the reader, with much to reflect on in this challenging and needed area of work.

Richard Bryant-Jefferies
June 2005

About the author

Richard Bryant-Jefferies qualified as a person-centred counsellor/therapist in 1994 and remains passionate about the application and effectiveness of this approach. Between early 1995 and mid-2003 Richard worked at a community drug and alcohol service in Surrey as an alcohol counsellor. Since 2003 he has worked for the Central and North West London Mental Health NHS Trust, managing substance misuse service within the Royal Borough of Kensington and Chelsea in London. He has experience of offering counselling and supervision in NHS, GP and private settings, and has provided training through 'alcohol awareness and response' workshops. He also offers workshops based on the use of written dialogue as a contribution to continuing professional development and within training programmes. His website address is www.bryant-jefferies. freeserve.co.uk

Richard had his first book on a counselling theme published in 2001, *Counselling the Person Beyond the Alcohol Problem* (Jessica Kingsley Publishers), providing theoretical yet practical insights into the application of the person-centred approach within the context of the 'cycle of change' model that has been widely adopted to describe the process of change in the field of addiction. Since then he has been writing for the *Living Therapy* series (Radcliffe Publishing), producing an on-going series of person-centred dialogues: *Problem Drinking, Time Limited Therapy in Primary Care, Counselling a Survivor of Child Sexual Abuse, Counselling a Recovering Drug User, Counselling Young People, Counselling for Progressive Disability, Relationship Counselling: sons and their mothers, Responding to a Serious Mental Health Problem, Person-Centred Counselling Supervision: personal and professional, Counselling for Obesity, Counselling for Eating Disorders in Men, Workplace Counselling in the NHS* and *Counselling for Problem Gambling*. The aim of the series is to bring the reader a direct experience of the counselling process, an exposure to the thoughts and feelings of both client and counsellor as they encounter each other on the therapeutic journey, and an insight into the value and importance of supervision.

Richard is also writing his first novel, 'Dying to Live', a story of traumatic loss, alcohol use and the therapeutic and has also adapted one of his books as a stage or radio play, and plans to do the same to other books in the series if the first is successful. However, he is currently seeking an opportunity for it to be recorded or staged.

Richard is keen to bring the experience of the therapeutic process, from the standpoint and application of the person-centred approach, to a wider audience. He is convinced that the principles and attitudinal values of this approach and the emphasis it places on the therapeutic relationship are key to helping people create greater authenticity both in themselves and in their lives, leading to a fuller and more satisfying human experience. By writing fictional accounts to try and bring the therapeutic process alive, to help readers engage with the characters within the narrative – client, counsellor and supervisor – he hopes to take the reader on a journey into the counselling room. Whether we think of it as pulling back the curtains or opening a door, it is about enabling people to access what can and does occur within the therapeutic process.

Acknowledgements

I wish to thank those who read through parts of the original draft and provided me with valuable feedback and comment: John Castle and David Jackson whose own military experiences contributed to my revising my first draft of the second part of this book to ensure greater authenticity; Menna Yarwood and Miriam Hollis for their forewords and valuable perspectives as person-centred counsellors working with clients seeking asylum from the effects of warfare and other forms of oppression.

I also wish to thank the Institute for War and Peace Reporting (IWPR Balkans) for permission to include the article by Belma Becirbasic and Dzenana Secic entitled: *Bosnia's raped women are being shunned by a society that refuses to see them as victims.*[1]

Once again I wish to express my appreciation to the team at Radcliffe Publishing for its support and commitment to the *Living Therapy* series.

---

[1] The goal of IWPR Balkans is 'to support the democratic transition of southeast Europe. The crisis in the Balkans is no longer military, but largely political and economic in nature. With many old institutions, practices and outlooks still in place, however, its painful transformation is in danger of stalling. New approaches, accommodations and solutions will have to be sought and promoted if the region is to develop economically and move forward towards European integration. Apart from some notable exceptions, media outlets and institutions are not yet providing consumers with clear analysis of the challenge for the region in the 21st century. The objective of IWPR in the Balkans is therefore to drive debate on these obstacles and milestones, and on the effect of international interventions and influence on the region'. From personal email correspondence with an IWPR Balkans representative. www.iwpr.net/balkans_index1.html

Introduction

The *Living Therapy* series aims to offer the reader an opportunity to experience and to appreciate, through the use of dialogue, some of the diverse and challenging issues that can arise during counselling. People remark on how readable these books are, how much they bring the therapeutic process alive and the timeliness of a series focusing on the application of the person-centred approach to working therapeutically with clients having specific issues. In particular, students of counselling and psychotherapy have commented on how accessible the text is. This is particularly heartening. I want the style to draw people into the narrative and feel engaged with the characters and the therapeutic process. I want this series to be what I would term 'an experiential read'.

As with the other titles in the *Living Therapy* (Radcliffe Publishing) series, this book is composed of fictitious dialogues between fictitious clients and their counsellors, and between their counsellors and their supervisors. Within the dialogues are woven the reflective thoughts and feelings of the clients, the counsellors and the supervisors, along with boxed comments on the process and references to person-centred theory.

Clearly the topic of warfare-induced psychological stress and trauma is a vast one. I do not seek to provide all the answers. Rather I want to convey something of the process of working with representative material that can arise so that the reader may be stimulated into processing their own reactions, and reflecting on the relevance and effectiveness of the therapeutic responses, and thereby gain insight into themselves and their practice. Often it will simply lead to more questions which I hope will prove stimulating to the reader and encourage them to think through their own theoretical, philosophical and ethical positions and their boundary of competence.

The dialogues

The book has been written to demonstrate the application of the person-centred approach (PCA) – a theoretical approach to counselling that has, at its heart, the power of the relational experience. It is this relational experience that I believe to be at the core of effective therapy, contributing to the possibility of releasing the client to realise greater potential for authentic living. The approach is widely used by counsellors working in the UK. In a membership survey in 2001 carried out by the British Association for Counselling and Psychotherapy, 35.6 per cent of those responding claimed to work to the person-centred approach, whilst 25.4 per cent identified themselves as psychodynamic practitioners.

If you have not read other titles in the *Living Therapy* series you may find it takes a while to adjust to the dialogue format. The responses offered by the counsellors, Debbie and Oliver, to their respective clients, Ania and Graham, are not to be read as simple reflections of the clients' words. Rather, the counsellors seek to voice empathic responses, often with a sense of 'checking out' that they are hearing accurately what the clients are saying. The client says something; the counsellor conveys what they have heard and senses the client is seeking to communicate to them, sometimes with the same words, sometimes with words that include a sense of what they feel is being communicated through the client's tone of voice, facial expression, or simply the relational atmosphere of the moment. The client is then enabled to confirm that she has been heard accurately, or correct the counsellor in her perception. The client may then explore more deeply what they have been saying or move on, in either case with a sense that they have been heard and warmly accepted. I have also included the inner thoughts and feelings that are present within the individuals who form the narrative.

The sessions are a little compressed. People will take different periods of time before choosing to disclose particular issues and working with their own process. This book is not intended to in any way indicate the length of time that may be needed to work with the kinds of issues that are addressed. The counsellor needs to be open and flexible to the needs of the client. For some clients, the process would take a lot longer. There are also clients who are ready to talk about difficult experiences almost immediately – their own organismic processes already driving memories, feelings, thoughts and experiences to the surface and into daily awareness.

In Part 1, the civilian victim of warfare is the focus. Ania, a refugee from Bosnia, describes her traumatic experiences and begins the process of addressing these in therapy. The counsellor is brought face-to-face with the reality of atrocity, rape, murder and violent death. She seeks to apply person-centred principles and practice in enabling her client to come to terms with what occurred for her. Memories are recovered, adding to the intensity of the experience for the client, and for the counsellor. The setting is a counselling centre that offers a service for people who are victims of torture and warfare.

In Part 2, Graham, ex-army, talks about his experiences and comes to terms with his feelings and memories. He describes his witnessing of the violent deaths of close comrades and of his own experience of killing, coming from a culture of 'men do not cry', and with little understanding of what counselling is, and certainly not something he would have ever expected to find himself on the receiving end of. The setting is a GP surgery. I have written elsewhere about the specific factors to consider when counselling in a GP surgery (Bryant-Jefferies, 2003b), for instance, time limited working, confidentiality and communication within a multi-disciplinary team, the setting itself and the culture of NHS healthcare (Bryant-Jefferies, 2005c) and attitudes towards counselling.

Supervision

Supervision sessions are included to offer the reader insight into the nature of therapeutic supervision in the context of the counselling profession, a method of supervising that I term 'collaborative review'. For many trainee counsellors, the use of supervision can be something of a mystery. This book contributes to unravelling this. I seek to demonstrate the application of the supervisory relationship. My intention is to show how supervision of the counsellor is very much a part of the process of enabling a client to work through issues.

Many professions do not recognise the need for some form of personal and process supervision, and often what is offered is line-management. However, counsellors are required to receive regular supervision in order to explore the dynamics of the relationship with their client, the impact of the work on the counsellor and their client, to receive support, to encourage professional development of the counsellor and to provide an opportunity for an experienced co-professional to monitor the supervisee's work in relation to ethical standards and codes of practice.

Supervision is an integral part of the therapeutic process. The sessions will help readers from other professions to recognise the value of supportive and collaborative supervision in order to help them become more authentically present with their own clients.

Merry, in discussing supervision, describes what he terms 'collaborative inquiry' as a 'form of research or inquiry in which two people (the supervisor and the counsellor) collaborate or co-operate in an effort to understand what is going on within the counselling relationship and within the counsellor'. He emphasises how this 'moves the emphasis away from "doing things right or wrong" (which seems to be the case in some approaches to supervision) to "how is the counsellor being, and how is that way of being contributing to the development of the counselling relationship based on the core conditions"' (Merry, 2002, p. 173). Elsewhere, Merry describes the relationship between person-centred supervision and congruence, indicating that 'a state of congruence . . . is the necessary condition for the therapist to experience empathic understanding and unconditional positive regard' (Merry, 2001, p. 183). Effective person-centred supervision provides a means through which congruence can be promoted within the therapist.

Tudor and Worrall (2004) have drawn together a number of theoretical and experiential strands from within and outside of the person-centred tradition in order to develop a theoretical position on the person-centred approach to supervision. This timely publication defines the necessary factors for effective supervision within this theoretical approach, and the respective responsibilities of both supervisor and supervisee in keeping with person-centred values and principles. They contrast person-centred working with other approaches to supervision and emphasise the importance of the therapeutic space as a place within which practitioners 'can dialogue freely between their personal philosophy and the philosophical assumptions which underlie their chosen theoretical orientation' (Tudor and Worrall, 2004, pp. 94–5). They affirm the values and attitudes of person-centred working and explore their application to the supervisory relationship.

It is the norm for all professionals working in the healthcare and social care environment in this age of regulation to be formally accredited or registered and to work to their own professional organisation's code of ethics or practice. Registered counselling practitioners with the British Association for Counselling and Psychotherapy are required to have regular supervision and continuing professional development to maintain registration. Whilst other professionals will gain much from this book in their work with clients experiencing the kind of issues here described, it is essential that they follow the standards, safeguards and ethical codes of their own professional organisation, and are appropriately trained and supervised to work with them on the issues that arise.

The person-centred approach (PCA)

The person-centred approach (PCA) was formulated by Carl Rogers and references are made to his ideas within the narrative of this book. For readers who are unfamiliar with this way of working we begin with an exploration of its theoretical base. Rogers proposed that certain conditions, when present within a therapeutic relationship, enable the client to develop towards what he termed 'fuller functionality'. Over a number of years he refined these ideas, which he defined as 'the necessary and sufficient conditions for constructive personality change'. These he described as:

1   Two persons are in psychological contact.
2   The first, whom we shall term the client, is in a state of incongruence, being vulnerable or anxious.
3   The second person, whom we shall term the therapist, is congruent or integrated in the relationship.
4   The therapist experiences unconditional positive regard for the client.
5   The therapist experiences an empathic understanding of the client's internal frame of reference and endeavours to communicate this experience to the client.
6   The communication to the client of the therapist's empathic understanding and unconditional positive regard is to a minimal degree achieved (Rogers, 1957, p. 96).

The first necessary and sufficient condition given for constructive personality change is that of 'two persons being in psychological contact'. However, although he later published this as simply 'contact' (Rogers, 1959) it is suggested (Wyatt and Sanders, 2002, p. 6) that this was written in 1953–4. They quote

Rogers as defining contact in the following terms: 'Two persons are in psychological contact, or have the minimum essential relationship when each makes a perceived or subceived difference in the experiential field of the other' (Rogers, 1959, p. 207). A recent exploration of the nature of psychological contact from a person-centred perspective is given by Warner (2002).

Contact

There is much to reflect on when considering a definition of 'contact' or 'psychological contact'. We could say that there is contact when the presence of the counsellor makes an impression, however small, on the field of awareness of the client. Is it a case of contact either being present or not, or is there is a kind of continuum with greater or lesser degrees of contact? It seems to me that it is both. Rather like the way that light may be regarded as either a particle or a wave, contact may be seen as a specific state of being, or as a process, depending upon what the perceiver is seeking to measure or observe. If I am trying to observe or measure whether there is contact, then my answer will be in terms of 'yes' or 'no'. If I am seeking to determine the degree to which contact exists, then the answer will be along a continuum. In other words, from the moment of minimal contact there is contact, and it can extend as more aspects of the client become present within the therapeutic relationship which, itself, may at times reach moments of increasing depth.

Empathy

Rogers defined empathy as meaning 'entering the private perceptual world of the other ... being sensitive, moment by moment, to the changing felt meanings which flow in this other person ... It means sensing meanings of which he or she is scarcely aware, but not trying to uncover totally unconscious feelings' (Rogers, 1980, p. 142). It is a very delicate process, and it provides a foundation block to effective person-centred therapy. The counsellor's role is primarily to establish empathic rapport and communicate empathic understanding to the client. This latter point is vital. Empathic understanding only has therapeutic value where it is communicated to the client.

   There is so much more to empathy than simply letting the client know what you understand from what they have communicated. It is also, and perhaps more significantly, the actual *process* of listening to a client, of attending – facial expression, body language, and presence – that is being offered and communicated and received *at the time that the client is speaking, at the time that the client is experiencing what is present for them.* It is, for the client, the knowing that, in the moment of an experience the counsellor is present and striving to be an understanding companion.

Unconditional positive regard

Within the therapeutic relationship the counsellor seeks to maintain an attitude of unconditional positive regard towards the client and all that they disclose. This is not 'agreeing with', it is simply warm acceptance of the fact that the client is being how they need or choose to be. Rogers wrote, 'when the therapist is experiencing a positive, acceptant attitude towards whatever the client *is* at that moment, therapeutic movement or change is more likely to occur' (Rogers, 1980, p. 116). Mearns and Thorne suggest that 'unconditional positive regard is the label given to the fundamental attitude of the person-centred counsellor towards her client. The counsellor who holds this attitude deeply values the humanity of her client and is not deflected in that valuing by any particular client behaviours. The attitude manifests itself in the counsellor's consistent acceptance of and enduring warmth towards her client' (Mearns and Thorne, 1988, p. 59).

Bozarth and Wilkins assert that 'unconditional positive regard is the curative factor in person-centred therapy' (Bozarth, 1998; Bozarth and Wilkins, 2001, p. vii). These two statements can be speculatively drawn together. We might then suggest that the unconditional positive regard experienced and conveyed by the counsellor, and received by the client, as an expression of the counsellor's valuing of their client's humanity, has a curative role in the therapeutic process. We might then add that this may be the case more specifically for those individuals who have been affected by a lack of unconditional warmth and prizing in their lives.

Congruence

Last, but by no means least, is that state of being that Rogers referred to as congruence, but which has also been described in terms of 'realness', 'transparency', 'genuineness' and 'authenticity'. Indeed Rogers wrote that '... genuineness, realness or congruence ... this means that the therapist is openly being the feelings and attitudes that are flowing within at the moment ... the term transparent catches the flavour of this condition' (Rogers, 1980, p. 115). Putting this into the therapeutic setting, we can say that 'congruence is the state of being of the counsellor when her outward responses to her client consistently match the inner feelings and sensations which she has in relation to her client' (Mearns and Thorne, 1999, p. 84). Interestingly, Rogers makes the following comment in his interview with Richard Evans that with regard to the three conditions, 'first, and most important, is therapist congruence or genuineness ... one description of what it means to be congruent in a given moment is to be aware of what's going on in your experiencing at that moment, to be acceptant towards that experience, to be able to voice it if it's appropriate, and to express it in some behavioural way' (Evans, 1975).

I would suggest that any congruent expression by the counsellor of their feelings or reactions has to emerge through the process of being in therapeutic relationship with the client. Indeed, the condition indicates that the therapist is 'congruent or integrated into the relationship'. This underlines the significance of the relationship. Being congruent is a disciplined way of being and not an open door to endless self-disclosure. Congruent expression is most appropriate and therapeutically valuable where it is informed by the existence of an empathic understanding of the client's inner world, and is offered in a climate of a genuine warm acceptance towards the client. Taking Rogers' comment quoted above regarding congruence as 'most important', we might suggest that unless the therapist is congruent in themselves and integrated in the relationship, then their empathy and unconditional positive regard would be at risk of not being authentic or genuine, and therefore having questionable therapeutic value.

Another view, however, is that it is in some way false to seek to separate out the three 'core conditions', that they exist together as a whole, mutually dependent on each others' presence in order to ensure that therapeutic relationship is established.

Perception

There is also the sixth condition, of which Rogers wrote: 'the final condition . . . is that the client perceives, to a minimal degree, the acceptance and empathy which the therapist experiences for him. Unless some communication of these attitudes has been achieved, then such attitudes do not exist in the relationship as far as the client is concerned, and the therapeutic process could not, by our hypothesis, be initiated' (Rogers, 1957). It is interesting that Rogers uses the words 'minimal degree', suggesting that the client does not need to fully perceive the fullness of the empathy and unconditional positive regard present within, and communicated by, the counsellor. A glimpse accurately heard and empathically understood is enough to have positive, therapeutic effect although logically one might think that the more that is perceived, the greater the therapeutic impact. But if it is a matter of intensity and accuracy, then a client experiencing a vitally important fragment of their inner world being empathically understood may be more significant to them, and more therapeutically significant, than a great deal being heard less accurately and with a weaker sense of therapist's understanding. The communication of the counsellor's empathy, congruence and unconditional positive regard, received by the client, creates the conditions for a process of constructive personality change.

Relationship is key

The PCA regards the relationship with clients, and the attitudes held within that relationship, to be key factors. In my experience, many adult psychological difficulties develop out of life experiences that involve problematic, conditional or abusive relational experiences. These can be centred in childhood or in later life, for example being a victim of warfare. What is significant is that the individual is left, through relationships that have a negative conditioning effect, affecting their perception of themselves and their potential as a person. Patterns are established in early life, bringing their own particular problems. However they can be exacerbated by conditional and psychologically damaging experiences later in life, that in some cases will have a resonance to what has occurred in the past, exacerbating the effects still further.

The result is a conditioned sense of self, with the individual thinking, feeling and acting in ways that enable them to maintain their self-beliefs and meanings within their learned or adapted concept of self. This is then lived out, the person seeking to satisfy what they have come to believe about themselves: needing to care either because it has been normalised, or in order to prove to themselves and the world that they are a 'good' person. They will need to maintain this conditioned sense of self and the sense of satisfaction that this gives them when it is lived out because they have developed such a strong identity with it.

Conditions of worth

The term, 'conditions of worth', applies to the conditioning mentioned earlier that is frequently present in childhood, and at other times in life, when a person experiences that their worth is conditional on their doing something, or behaving, in a certain way. This is usually to satisfy someone else's needs, and can be contrary to the client's own sense of what would be a satisfying experience. The values of others become a feature of the individual's structure of self. The person moves away from being true to themselves, learning instead to remain 'true' to their conditioned sense of worth. This state of being in the client is challenged by the person-centred therapist by offering them unconditional positive regard and warm acceptance. These therapeutic attitudes provide what may be a new experience or one that in the past the client has dismissed, preferring to stay with that which matches and therefore reinforces their conditioned sense of worth and sense of self.

Offering someone a non-judgemental, warm, accepting and authentic relationship – (perhaps a kind of 'therapeutic love') – provides an opportunity to grow into a fresh sense of self in which their potential as a person can be fulfilled. Such an experience can enable the client to redefine themselves as they experience the presence of the therapist's congruence, empathy and unconditional positive regard. This process can take time. Often the personality change that is required to sustain a shift away from what have been termed 'conditions of worth' may require a lengthy period of therapeutic work, bearing in mind that the person may be struggling to unravel a sense of self that has been developed, sustained and reinforced for many decades of life.

Unconditional positive regard and warm acceptance offered consistently over time can, and does, enable clients to begin to question their beliefs about themselves and to begin to build into their structure of self the capacity to see and experience themselves as being of value for who they are. It enables them to liberate themselves from the constraints of patterns of conditioning.

Actualising tendency

A crucial feature or factor in this process of 'constructive personality change' is the presence of what Rogers termed 'the actualising tendency'; a tendency towards fuller and more complete personhood with an associated greater fulfilment of their potentialities. The role of the person-centred counsellor is to provide the facilitative climate within which this tendency can work constructively. The 'therapist trusts the actualizing tendency of the client and truly believes that the client who experiences the freedom of a fostering psychological climate will resolve his or her own problems' (Bozarth, 1998, p. 4). This is fundamental to the application of the PCA. Rogers wrote: 'the person-centred approach is built on a basic trust in the person ... (It) depends on the actualizing tendency present in every living organism – the tendency to grow, to develop, to realize its full potential. This way of being trusts the constructive directional flow of the human-being towards a more complex and complete development. It is this directional flow that we aim to release' (Rogers, 1986, p. 198).

For some people, at certain stages, rather than producing a liberating experience, there will instead be a tendency to maintain the status quo, perhaps a fear of change, uncertainty, or the implications of change are such that the person prefers to maintain the known, the certain. In a sense, there is a liberation from the imperative to change and grow which may bring temporary – and perhaps permanent – relief for the person. The actualising tendency may work through the part of the person that needs relief from change, enhancing its presence for the period of time that the person experiences a need to maintain this. The person-centred therapist will not try to move the person from this place or state. It is to be accepted, warmly and unconditionally. And, of course, sometimes in the moment of acceptance the person is enabled to question whether that really is how they want to be.

Configurations within self

Configurations within self (Mearns and Thorne, 2000) are discrete sets of thoughts, feelings and behaviours that develop through the experience of life. They emerge in response to a range of experiences, including the process of introjection and the symbolisation of experiences and dissonant self-experience within the person's structure of self. They can also exist in what Mearns terms as ' "growthful" and "not for growth", configurations' (Mearns and Thorne, 2000, pp. 114–16), each offering a focus for the actualising tendency, the former seeking an expansion into new areas of experience with all that that brings; the latter seeking to energise the status quo and to block change because of its potential for disrupting the current order within the structure of self. The actualising tendency may not always manifest through growth or developmental change. It can also manifest through periods of stabilisation and stability, of denial to experience. During the counselling process, as the client gains fuller contact with his or her own experience, and develops a greater sense of trust towards the counsellor, they will be encouraged to voice and explore this, drawing it into the open, into awareness, from which it can be more effectively worked with, and perhaps re-defined in a different way.

Mearns suggests that these 'parts' or 'configurations' interrelate 'like a family, with an individual variety of dynamics'. As within any 'system', change in one area will impact on the functioning of the system. Mearns therefore comments that 'when the interrelationship of configurations changes, it is not that we are left with something entirely new: we have the same "parts" as before, but some which may have been subservient before are stronger, others which were judged adversely are accepted, some which were in self-negating conflict have come to respect each other, and overall the parts have achieved constructive integration with the energy release which arises from such fusion' (Mearns, 1999, pp. 147–8). The growing acceptance of the configurations, their own fluidity and movement within the self-structure and the increased, open and more accurate communication between the parts, is, perhaps, another way of considering the integrating of the threads of experience to which Rogers refers.

Understanding the configurational nature of ourselves enables us to understand why we are triggered into certain thoughts, feelings and behaviours, and how they group together, serving a particular experiential purpose for the person. From this theoretical perspective we can argue that the person-centred counsellor's role is essentially facilitative. It creates the therapeutic climate of empathic understanding, unconditional positive regard and authenticity building up a relational climate that encourages the client to move into a more fluid state with more openness to their own experience and the discovery of a capacity towards a fuller actualising of their potential.

In another title in this series I used the analogy of treating a wilting plant (Bryant-Jefferies, 2003b, p. 12). The plant can be sprayed with a specific herbicide or pesticide to eradicate a perceived disease that may be present in it, and that may be enough. But perhaps the true cause of the disease is that the plant is located in harsh surroundings; for example too much sun and not enough water, poor soil and near to other plants that it finds difficulty in surviving so close to. Maybe by offering the plant a healthier environment that will facilitate greater nourishment according to the needs of the plant, it may become the strong, healthy plant it has the potential to become. Yes, the chemical intervention may also be helpful, but if the true causes of the diseases are environmental – essentially the plant's relationship with that which surrounds it – then it won't achieve sustainable growth. We may not be able to transplant it, but we can provide water, nutrients and maybe shade from a fierce sun. Therapy, it seems to me, exists to provide this healthy environment within which the 'wilting' client can begin the process of receiving the nourishment (in the form of healthy relational experience) that can enable them, in time, to become a more fully functioning person.

Relationship re-emphasised

In addressing these factors the therapeutic relationship is central. A therapeutic approach such as the person-centred one affirms that it is not what you do so much as *how you are* with your client that is therapeutically significant, and this 'how you are' has to be received by the client. Gaylin highlights the importance of client perception. 'If clients believe that their therapist is working on their behalf – if they perceive caring and understanding – then therapy is likely to be successful. It is the condition of attachment and the perception of connection that have the power to release the faltered actualization of the self.' He goes on to stress how 'we all need to feel connected, prized – loved', describing human-beings as 'a species born into mutual interdependence', and that there 'can be no self outside the context of others. Loneliness is de-humanizing and isolation anathema to the human condition. The relationship,' he suggests 'is what psychotherapy is all about' (Gaylin, 2001, p. 103).

Love is an important word though not necessarily one often used to describe therapeutic relationship. Patterson, however, gives a valuable definition of love as it applies to the person-centred therapeutic process. He writes, 'we define love as an attitude that is expressed through empathic understanding, respect and compassion, acceptance, and therapeutic genuineness, or honesty and openness towards others' (Patterson, 2000, p. 315). We all need love, but most of all we need it during our developmental period of life. He also affirms that 'whilst love is important throughout life for the well-being of the individual, it is particularly important, indeed absolutely necessary, for the survival of the infant and for providing the basis for the normal psychological development of the individual' (Patterson, 2000, pp. 314–5).

When working with refugees who are victims of warfare the therapeutic emphasis needs, in particular, to be strongly placed on the sense of 'prizing' and 'valuing' of the client. The counsellor needs to experience and convey that they are 'really very interested in what may be going on for the client', and that they 'genuinely care about them in the process of working their way through it' (Hollis, 2004). A very human experience arises, helping the client to begin to feel the possibility of some degree of certainty and reassurance in what is likely to be a very uncertain situation. This quality of human-to-human reassurance becomes an important factor in the relationship-building process.

Process of change from a person-centred perspective

Rogers was interested in understanding the process of change, what it was like, how it occurred and what experiences it brought to those involved – client and therapist. At different points he explored this. Embleton Tudor *et al.* (2004) point to a model consisting of 12 steps identified in 1942 by Rogers and to his two later chapters on this topic (Rogers, 1951), and finally the seven-stage model (1958/1967). Roges wrote of 'initially looking for elements which would mark or characterize change itself'. However, what he experienced from his enquiry and research into the process of change he summarised as: 'individuals move, I began to see, not from fixity or homeostasis through change to a new fixity, though such a process is indeed possible. But much the more significant continuum is from fixity to changingness, from rigid structure to flow, from stasis to process. I formed the tentative hypothesis that perhaps the qualities of the client's expression at any one point might indicate his position on this continuum, where he stood in the process of change' (Rogers, 1967, p. 131).

Change, then, involves a movement from fixity to greater fluidity, from, we might say, a rigid set of attitudes and behaviours to a greater openness to experience, to variety and diversity. Change might be seen as having a certain liberating quality, a freeing up of the human-being – his heart, mind, emotions – so that the person experiences themselves less a fixed object and more of a conscious process. The list below is taken from Rogers' summary of the process, indicating the changes that people will show.

1   This process involves a loosening of feelings.
2   This process involves a change in the manner of experiencing.
3   The process involves a shift from incongruence to congruence.
4   The process involves a change in the manner in which, and the extent to which the individual is able and willing to communicate himself in a receptive climate.
5   The process involves a loosening of the cognitive maps of experience.
6   There is a change in the individual's relationship to his problem.
7   There is a change in the individual's manner of relating (Rogers, 1967, pp. 156–8).

This is a brief overview; the chapter in which Rogers describes the process of change has much more detail and should be read in order to gain a clear grasp not only of the process as a whole, but of the distinctive features of each stage (Rogers, 1967, pp. 132–55). Embleton Tudor *et al.* summarise this process in the helpful terms: 'a movement from fixity to fluidity, from closed to open, from tight to loose, and from afraid to accepting' (Embleton Tudor *et al.*, 2004, p. 47).

Rogers points out that there are several types of process by which personality changes and that the one he describes is 'set in motion when the individual experiences himself as being fully received'. Does this process apply to all psychotherapies? Rogers indicates that more data are needed, adding that 'perhaps therapeutic approaches which place great stress on the cognitive and little on the emotional aspects of experience may set in motion an entirely different process of change'. In terms of whether this process of change would generally be viewed as desirable and that it would move the person in a valued direction, Rogers expresses the view that the valuing of a particular process of change was linked to social value judgements made by individuals and cultures. He points out that the process of change that he described could be avoided, simply by people 'reducing or avoiding those relationships in which the individual is fully received as he is' (Rogers, 1967, p. 155).

Rogers also takes the view that change is unlikely to be rapid; many clients enter the therapeutic process at stage two, and leave at stage four, having during that period gained enough to feel satisfied. He suggested it would be 'very rare, if ever, that a client who fully exemplified stage one would move to a point where he fully exemplified stage seven', and that if this did occur 'it would involve a matter of years' (Rogers, 1967, pp. 155–6). At the outset, threads of experience are discerned and understood separately by the client but as the process of change takes place, they move into 'the flowing peak moments of therapy in which all these threads become inseparably woven together.' Rogers continues: 'in the new experiencing with immediacy which occurs at such moments, feeling and cognition interpenetrate, self is subjectively present in the experience, volition is simply the subjective following of a harmonious balance of organismic direction. Thus, as the process reaches this point the person becomes a unity of flow, of motion. He has changed, but what seems most significant, he has become an integrated process of changingness' (Rogers, 1967, p. 158).

It conjures up images of flowing movement, perhaps we should say purposeful flowing movement as being the essence of the human condition, a state that we each have the potential to become, or to realise. Is it something we generate or develop out of fixity, or does it exist within us all as a potential that we lose during our conditional experiencing in childhood? Are we discovering something new, or re-discovering something that was lost?

Responding to trauma

Diagnosis

Before we can discuss responses to trauma, we have to consider the acceptability of the term from a person-centred perspective. People are diagnosed as having been traumatised, or as suffering from 'post-traumatic stress disorder' (PTSD). The PCA, however, questions the helpfulness and, indeed, the validity of the diagnostic process. I have referred elsewhere (Bryant-Jefferies, 2003b) to the debate as to whether diagnosis can necessarily be trusted and empirical when it comes to mental health factors, drawing attention to Bozarth (2002) who refers to his own studies of particular diagnostic concepts which do not evidence the clustering of symptoms in a meaningful way (Bozarth, 1998) and to those of others in relation to schizophrenia (Bentall, 1990; Slade and Cooper, 1979), depression (Hallett, 1990; Wiener, 1989), agoraphobia (Hallam, 1983), borderline personality-disorder (Kutchins and Kirk, 1997) and panic disorder (Hallam, 1989).

Rogers also questioned the value of psychological diagnosis. He argued that it could place the client's locus of value firmly outside themselves and definitely within the diagnosing 'expert', leaving the client at risk of developing tendencies of dependence and expectation that the 'expert' will have the responsibility of improving the client's situation (Rogers, 1951, p. 223). It has been the custom to respond to trauma by providing counsellors, therapists and psychologists to help people to de-brief, process and minimise the psychological damage caused by severe trauma, for example that experienced in war situations. Typical experiences are extreme violence, extreme loss and constant fear and terror. The idea has been that by helping people work through the experience they can enable them to re-process what has happened to them in such a way that the psychological phenomena labelled PTSD can be minimised.

However, this has been questioned by Bracken and Petty (1998) who suggest that the exporting of models developed within the context of Western psychiatry may not necessarily be the most appropriate for all cultures. They draw together a range of contributors with experience of working in the field who have been involved in helping adults and children to rebuild their lives after witnessing the destruction of families and communities.

Of course, the person-centred approach is itself a model generated from within Western society, although in many ways it remains a radical departure from the directive, expert led interventions that typify most psychiatric and psychological responses. It seems to me that the essential humanity of the person-centred approach; the values, the belief in the potential of persons to have resources within themselves that can be tapped to enable them to come through traumatic experiencing, are elements that have global application. My hope and expectation would be that a person-centred counsellor, by virtue of the discipline and philosophy of the approach, would be working in a way that is empathically sensitive towards, and warmly accepting of, cultural difference and the diverse cultural methods of dealing with traumatic experiencing.

However, it has to be stated that not everyone is traumatised by trauma. Trauma is an event but the process of being traumatised does not necessarily follow. It depends on how the individual reacts, how they regard what has happened, how much resilience they have to the psychological impact of what has occurred. Not everyone evidences all the symptoms categorised under PTSD. The actual diagnosis can set up an expectation in the client – and the counsellor – as to what is being and may be experienced. But there is no guarantee that this will be the case. The danger is that by making general reference to 'the traumatised client', a set of expectations and assumptions are made, and the individuality and uniqueness of the person is lost. This is not acceptable to the person-centred approach that values – prizes – the individuality of the person and their uniqueness in responding to and dealing with events in their lives.

In this book the literature regarding the different theoretical responses to extreme trauma are not reviewed, but rather the focus is on how a person-centred therapist responds and what theoretical perspective their responding is based on.

Loss and trauma

It is my view that some victims of warfare and conflict can lose something very precious in the process of their traumatising experience, or perhaps I should say receive something, the effect of which is this loss. By this I mean the direct experience and therefore intimate knowledge of the destructive capacity of the human-being, and its ability to inflict pain and suffering on others, and in particular the known reality that it can happen to them and/or to those they are closest to – family, friends, colleagues and comrades-in-arms. For some this experience will change the way that they view people. Something becomes known, not as an intellectual piece of knowledge – something read in the papers – but it is an actual, real experience. The individual *knows* how fellow human-beings can act towards one another, people who, as is often the case, will have been living side by side with each other. There is something about this knowing of the capacity of the human-being to inflict pain and suffering that has a significantly traumatising effect. It is as though the victim has been brought face-to-face with an aspect of the reality of the human-being that many people do not ever experience. In a sense the victim of warfare, torture, atrocity, repression has a wider experience of the reality of human potential, or at least, one aspect of it. Through the experience it is possible to lose sight of the essential humanity that is also present in persons, though clearly it has been lost sight of by the perpetrator of personal violence.

What can a person-centred counsellor or psychotherapist offer a person who has been traumatised by loss of their family and community, by violence upon themselves and those close to them? How can that person begin the process of surviving psychologically? To me it seems that it comes back to our sense of humanity. This may not seem like a very technical term in the context of the psychology of the person, but when you are faced with a person who has experienced the worst kinds of conflict, the worst kinds of loss, the worst and most gruesome experiences of physical harm, there are no comforting words because the experience is beyond comforting. They are what they are – acts of inhumanity perpetrated upon another. And they therefore, if congruence is to be achieved, need to be seen and known for what they are. Therefore, the counsellor working with the victim must be able to accept that in the moment of sitting with them all that they have to offer is themselves as a fellow human-being, prepared to be open to the horror that is present within the client. And until we have sat with someone who *knows* the capacity of human-beings to inflict pain, who *knows* the depth of physical, emotional and mental pain that can arise in situations of war, we cannot be totally sure just how we will react. Working in this area takes the counsellor to an edge, in fact beyond an edge, that edge of awareness and experience that they have previously known. I also mention this 'edge' in relation to psychosis elsewhere (Bryant-Jefferies, 2005a; b). The need for supervision to enable the counsellor to work at and beyond this edge, if you like beyond their previous horizon of human experience and awareness, is demanding and disorientating, deeply affecting and potentially produces in the therapist experiences that in some way parallel those of the client. They too are being brought face-to-face with aspects of being human and of the human experience that confront and challenge their own philosophy of life, their own structure of belief as to what it means to be a person. Supervision is necessary to ensure that the impact of the therapeutic process does not disrupt the counsellor's congruence, and where it does, the offering of the core conditions in supervision will facilitate the therapist in exploring and resolving what has developed.

The person-centred counsellor is working to a philosophy and theoretical discipline that prizes the human person, that seeks to offer clients a set of relational experiences that will create a relational climate in which constructive personality change can occur. A client who has been psychologically affected within a war zone can enter an intensely individual and isolating experiential world. They need to be invited (not forced) back into human relationship.

The blitzkrieg

Thinking back to the blitz in London in the Second World War, many people lost friends, family, homes and watched the structure of their communities reduced to rubble. What helped people to survive this psychologically? I would suggest family and community, the sense of solidarity that can emerge among people who face a collective enemy. We perhaps see this today in the response of people in Iraq to the bombing they have had to endure, families coming together, people grouping in solidarity around cultural and religious beliefs.

But in many war zones today it is often the community that is destroyed, people can become isolated, scattered, as they flee for their lives. They are surely at greater risk of psychological difficulties as a result. The need to bring people together and to foster that sense of community and solidarity seems a vital part of the process of rehabilitation.

There is also the factor that perhaps in some parts of the world, or at particular periods in history, there exists a strong sense of 'getting on with it'. I spoke to Peggy Simmons (née Cocks) who, as a member of the WAAF, had a leg blown off after an enemy plane jettisoned its bomb load near where she was walking near Victoria Station in the Second World War. She writes on a BBC website of her experience,[1] 'I was hit by part of a bomb and lost my left leg. There was no pain – I can remember people asking me the phone number of my next of kin which I gave them. I did not lose consciousness. I nearly died, loss of blood, etc. I was taken to Westminster Hospital where I remained for four weeks.' She cites the support and encouragement she received, in particular her parents, and how she relearned 'to cycle, ride a horse, drive, dance, swim, sail and canoe. Later I did rock climbing and abseiling.' She also returned to her job as a driver. There was no counselling as we understand it, and she experienced no need for it.

---

[1] www.bbc.co.uk/dna/ww2/A2691867

It happened, and she got on with her life. How different she was as a result of the event is hard to quantify, but she is not aware of it as having had a psychologically disabling effect.

But someone else may have reacted differently, internalising the experience in a different way. Or perhaps a different person may have had less familial support, or less opportunity to engage in activities that would contribute to their psychological well-being and self-confidence. With warfare causing an increasingly higher percentage of civilian casualties compared to military personnel, there may often not be family members alive. Perhaps there is also something about seeing horrifying events occurring to others that makes a deeper impact, at least for some people. But maybe not everyone. Again, we have to be careful not to imagine that everyone who experiences trauma is traumatised, or in a way consistent with a particular understanding of what it means.

Psychological breakdown

Rogers wrote of the process of psychological breakdown and disorganisation. He expressed four stages to this process, the first two stages of which 'may be illustrated by anxiety-producing experiences in therapy, or by acute psychotic breakdowns'.

'If the individual has a large or significant degree of *incongruence between self and experience* and if a significant experience demonstrating this *incongruence* occurs suddenly, or with a high degree of obviousness, then the organism's process of *defense* is unable to operate successfully.

'As a result *anxiety is experienced*, as the *incongruence* is subceived. The degree of anxiety is dependent upon the extent of the *self-structure* which is *threatened*' (Rogers, 1959, pp. 228–9).

As a result of this process Rogers then went on to describe the effects this has on the individual's self-structure and subsequent bahaviour, as follows.

'The process of defense being unsuccessful, the *experience* is *accurately symbolised* in *awareness*, and the gestalt of the *self-structure* is broken by this *experience* of the *incongruence* in *awareness*. A state of disorganisation results.

'In such a state of disorganisation the organism behaves at times in ways which are openly consistent with experiences which have hitherto been distorted or denied to awareness. At other times the self may temporarily regain regnancy, and the organism may behave in ways consistent with it. Thus in such a state of disorganisation, the tension between the concept of self (with its included distorted perceptions) and the experiences which are not accurately symbolised or included in the concept of self, is expressed in a confused regnancy, first one and then the other supplying the "feedback" by which the organism regulates behaviour' (Rogers, 1959, p. 229).

Joseph (2003) links this to the phenomenon of PTSD and uses this to describe a person-centred theoretical view of the psychological process that leads to PTSD and the significance of the person-centred therapy as an effective approach in enabling clients to resolve what has occurred. He acknowledges that person-centred therapists do not take the view that there are specific treatments for specific disorders and that 'psychopathology develops as a result of the internalization of conditions of worth creating an incongruence between self and experience, and so a therapeutic environment characterized by unconditional positive regard will be healing because it serves to dissolve the client's conditions of worth' (Joseph, 2003, p. 70), citing Bozarth (1998). He then refers to Purton (2002) in questioning whether all psychological disturbances arise out of the introjection of conditional regard, citing a car accident as an example that left a client with symptoms of PTSD.

The importance of the particular and personal meaning that the individual internalises as a result of an experience, and the effect that this has on their accepted view of themselves and of the world is key. Joseph, in the same paper, draws from the work of Janoff-Bulman (1992) with regard to how people have assumptive worlds, and that the sudden experience of a traumatic event can shatter them. He draws attention to her idea of there being three core assumptions: that the world is benevolent, that the world is meaningful, and that the self is worthy. Unless early life experiences have disrupted this view, most people do, indeed, live on a day-to-day basis in line with these assumptions.

But some traumatic event, for example, a situation that arises within a war zone where a person is exposed to atrocity, or is themselves the subject of torture, rape, the destruction of their family and community, then the effect can be to shatter these assumptions, where they are present. The person now has immediate and intensely personal knowledge, charged with emotion and feeling, that reality is different, people can be different, and he or she can be a victim of the worst kinds of inhumanity. The new information can only be in some way ignored and rejected, or assimilated. In that experience, the structure of self can break down if it cannot – or will not – accept the reality of what has occurred. People are then left to act out of a state of inner disorganisation. Behaviours emerge that may seem hard to explain from the outside, but are perfectly reasonable attempts to deal with what has happened for the affected person. Traumatic impact on a person's structure of self can also take people into a specific state or place within themselves, a discrete identity within the person's structure of self that is created to hold and perhaps contain what has been, or is being, experienced. They may then find themselves dwelling in this part that has been violently generated for a short or longer period of time. This 'part' has in a sense been imposed upon the person's functioning structure of self. The self-structure as it was remains, but this new element may hold a dominant position, requiring adjustment. Or it may get buried in order to contain its potentially devastating impact on the rest of the system. It is possible that in some instances, this 'part' may contain memories of experiences that remain hidden from usual daily awareness, perhaps providing the basis for a form of dissociative experiencing. These memories may then later erupt into awareness either within or outside of the therapeutic process.

Joseph (2003, p. 73) offers the following process based on Rogers' ideas in his 1959 paper.

Traumatic event that is sudden, obvious and demonstrates incongruence
between self and experience

↓

Breakdown and disorganisation of self-structure

↓

Phenomenology typical of post-traumatic stress
(intrusive and avoidant experiences)

↓

Person-centred therapy

↓

Client accurately symbolises in awareness their experience

↓

Reintegration of self and experience in a way consistent with
actualising tendency

↓

Post-traumatic stress diminishes

↓

Become more fully functioning

↓

Phenomenology typical of post-traumatic growth

The key is that the person-centred therapist at the core of their therapeutic methodology is offering the environment in which a client's incongruence can emerge more fully into awareness. Added to this, they are working towards greater congruence within the client as the experience is integrated and the client's structure of self adjusts and evolves. As a result, greater congruence emerges as the client's self-concept develops anew in response to the process taking place, post-traumatic stress diminishes as a disabling feature within the client's life and awareness, and what has been termed 'post-traumatic growth', is evidenced.

Post-traumatic growth

'Post-traumatic growth refers to positive changes following trauma, and it is reported that between 30 and 90 per cent of survivors report at least some positive changes following trauma' (Linley and Joseph, 2002, p. 14). In their article cited above, the authors conclude that this phenomenon is 'typically reported in three broad domains of closer relationships, improved perceptions of self, and changed philosophies of life' (Linley and Joseph, 2002, p. 17). If, as evidence suggests, traumatic experience can induce an experience of 'growth', then we are perhaps reminded of the Chinese glyph for 'crisis' that, I understand, is made up of the glyphs for 'danger' and 'opportunity'. Perhaps we might redefine psychological trauma as being 'crises presenting opportunity in the presence of danger'.

From a person-centred perspective, this is an interesting debate, given the core acceptance of the actualising tendency. Although whether this should be defined as a 'growthful' tendency is itself a matter of debate. As mentioned earlier, Mearns (Mearns and Thorne, 2000, pp. 114–16) writes of 'growthful' and 'not-for-growth' configurations within the self. Given traumatic experience there may be aspects of the structure of self that will want to say 'enough is enough', 'no more', 'overload' and 'I just want to hide away for a while'. These need to be heard and offered the same quality of unconditional positive regard as those parts of the person that seem to be more expansive and developmental, progressive, if you like, and taking the person towards new experiences. The psyche is a system of checks and balances, with parts working together to generate the most productive outcome that satisfies the needs of the person. Sometimes the need to stop outweighs the need to keep going. Working with traumatic experience can involve hearing that call to stop, and also a reassessment of the experiential situation, a reintegration of the structure of self, a redefinition of the self-concept, and then where possible a moving on. Putting aside for a moment the debate around how we define post-traumatic stress disorder, and how it should be treated, the experience is intense and can be deep-seated with many protective psychological barriers erected to protect the individual from the effects of their experience, or simply to enable them to cope and to survive. The person-centred counsellor or therapist will trust the client's process and timing and will not seek to break down any protective factors. Their role will be to provide the therapeutic conditions, the therapeutic relationship, and therefore the opportunity for constructive personality change, whatever form it takes for the individual concerned.

Conclusion

The person-centred therapist has a perfectly adequate theoretical basis from which to work with clients who have been seriously psychologically affected by events and experiences that have disrupted their structure of self and brought into question their self-concept. The person-centred counsellor seeks to form therapeutic relationships with their client. What is it that is therapeutically helpful about this relationship? What does the person who is experiencing, or has experienced a traumatising event, really want? What are they screaming out for from the core of their being, though they may not always be aware of this inner scream? Perhaps to be reassured that there are people who care, who, though they cannot genuinely understand what has been experienced, are willing and ready to be beside them as they try to make sense of their shattered world, and often shattered structure of self.

This latter point is crucially important when considering working with people for whom experiences in adult life have had a traumatising effect, or for whom these experiences have occurred at a time after they have established their structure of self, and within this, their self-concept. However, we should not lose sight of the fact that many, many children and young people are psychologically affected by the trauma of warfare, with the likelihood that many children will develop dissociative and fragile states (Warner, 2000) in response, severely affecting the development of their structure of self.

The offering of the core conditions, the trusting of the timeliness of the client seeking help, the acknowledgement and attempt to work with the actualising tendency within the person, all contribute to the relevance and application of the person-centred approach to working with victims of trauma as a result, for instance, of warfare.

The military experience

The psychological impact of war-related trauma on the soldier has been the subject of much study. Palmer (2002) in his chapter exploring 'psychotherapy, the psychology of trauma and army psychiatry since 1904' refers to seven studies across the twentieth century (Ahrenfeld, 1958; Binneveld, 1997; Culpin, 1920; Myers, 1940; Rivers, 1916, 1918; Shephard, 2000). He stresses the importance of the bonding between comrades in arms, with the resulting effect that, as highlighted in Western military literature, soldiers will fight for each other rather than for a particular cause. As a result, when death is suffered amongst their number, there will be the experience of grief. He goes on to highlight a number of areas of grief and loss: 'death of friends and the maiming of comrades or self', and the way the loss may be magnified 'by a loss of faith in the system and the loss of control of their lives for a period of time with the concomitant feelings of helplessness and the experience of near death' (Palmer, 2002, p. 228).

Palmer lists the following psychological reactions to combat.

- *During combat*: acute stress reactions (ASRs).
- *After combat*: post-traumatic stress reactions (PTSRs), post-traumatic mental illness (PTMI) – depression, anxiety, phobias, PTSD, post-conflict syndromes (PCSs) and substance abuse (Palmer, 2002, p. 237).

Obviously, there is a need for a range of medical and psychological interventions, however, Palmer also points to the strong sense of 'group' within the armed forces, highlighting the role of the Regimental tradition, the possibility of family members who have been in the Regiment or Armed Forces. Fighting units are small. The Army has a buddy system where personnel are trained to fight in pairs with each looking after the other in action. Groups of buddies are then formed into Sections, and Sections then form Platoons that are normally the smallest fighting unit as a group under fighting conditions. It is a tight and disciplined set of organised relationships designed to ensure maximum effectiveness.

Palmer suggests that 'Junior and Senior NCOs, Regimental Sergeant Majors and Officers may', and in his opinion 'should, be much more important than most mental health personnel' (Palmer, 2002, p. 229). The Regiment is a 'family' and provides support for both military personnel and their families. We might view the military environment, the roles, the relationships that have been generated, as protective factors that can minimise the impact of traumatic experiencing, providing an environment in which the individual can be managed and most effectively rehabilitated. It is interesting that in some ways this parallels the idea of protective factors within families where a child's upbringing is disrupted by, for instance, parental behaviour stemming from alcohol misuse – the idea that the formation and strengthening of other familial relationships (with aunts, uncles or grandparents, for example), or perhaps relationships with teachers or neighbours, can help to minimise the damaging effect (Velleman, 2001).

There is another view that might go some way to explain a certain degree of resilience within military personnel to the psychological trauma than can arise in combat situations. Going back to Rogers' ideas regarding psychological breakdown (Rogers, 1959), and Janoff-Bulman's (1992) ideas regarding the shattering of core assumptions in the face of traumatic experiencing, it could be that the preparation of military personnel for combat is in part a process of reorganising the core assumptions, re-patterning, if you like, the person's structure of self such that the exposure to loss, atrocity, violent death and intense threat is less shattering. In other words, if these experiences – or the possibility of these experiences – have become to some degree symbolised in awareness and accepted, then perhaps their appearance in reality may be less shattering on the individual's structure of self. I say maybe. The hypothesis that a person can be, if you like, re-configured to accept experiences that would shatter other people psychologically seems reasonable. And it would explain, as well, why some people may find it so difficult to adjust away from that re-configuring at the end of a military career.

Barrett-Lennard has commented on Rogers' work with returning war veterans and his commitment to the development of counselling resources for them towards the end of the Second World War. He highlights that 'besides the emotional legacies of combat itself, a core issue is the difficult transition from a highly organized, structurally authoritative military system to a fluidly undefined (relatively non-directive) peacetime democracy (Barrett-Lennard, 1998, p. 53). Elsewhere he refers to a paper by Rogers, 'Psychological adjustments of discharged service personnel', commenting that 'the personal difficulties given special and vivid attention by Rogers included the frequent deep anger and pent-up hostilities of returning veterans; disturbances to self-esteem which a diagnostic approach to helping quite often exacerbated; a frequent loss of purpose in the more amorphous civilian context; a wide range of distressing problems in marriage and family relations; and the hardships of learning to live with physical handicap' (Barrett-Lennard, 1998, p. 50).

It should also be commented on that the person who joins the military does not do so with the thought or the intention of experiencing life as a war veteran. People choose a military career path for many reasons, but the consequences of that choice in terms of the effects of warfare and combat are not something that the person is truly prepared for. Yes, prepared for coping whilst within the military context, but outside of that, and particularly when suffering from the physical, emotional and mental scars of combat, this is not something that can be prepared for. It is not planned for on the military career path. This is an aspect of the military experience for the counsellor to have empathy for. The military person has chosen to serve their country in a particular way and, in effect, to put their lives in the hands of others. They do not need prejudicial and judgemental attitudes from peace-loving therapists. The war veteran does need honest, matter-of-fact, person-to-person relationship. The importance of getting the relationship right cannot be stressed enough.

Further thoughts

I want to add something drawn from my comments above in relation to other cultural expectations and how they may have shaped a person's self-structure and self-concept. Do the core assumptions made by Janoff-Bulman really have universal application? If you are brought up in, for instance, a refugee camp where, perhaps, you feel constantly under threat, or you live your life in a society constantly under a very real and believable threat from bomb outrages, is it not highly likely that you could have very different core assumptions? Or if your early life was shaped in an oppressive society where violence, torture and 'disappearance' were commonplace, would you not have developed very different assumptions based on the reality of experience? And therefore, might not the impact be different in some way? Might the shattering of the self-structure be less (or different – I do not want to minimise the significance of the act, merely the impact on the person) because the event that occurred is one that has been accepted as possible and, to some degree, lived with as a likelihood on a day-to-day, hour-by-hour basis? I want to reiterate that when working at the human 'edge' we have only our humanity to offer. And in saying this, I don't want to say 'only', because I believe that the humanity that an individual can carry into relationship extends to depths of being beyond normal everyday awareness and experience. For me, the excitement – is that the right word? – of the therapeutic movement is that it is opening up a new frontier, the exploration of inner space, of the human experience and, perhaps most important, the significance of human relationship both as a potentially damaging but also as a healing and developmental factor. For me there is something about the human heart, the quality of heartfelt response, that carries something significant for the world of counselling and psychotherapy, and I believe this is very much at the heart of the person-centred approach. I do not think we have, as yet, paid enough attention on the qualities of the heart as factors in the process of therapeutic work.

Developments in PCA

I am extremely encouraged by the increasing interest in the person-centred approach, the growing amount of material being published, and the realisation that relationship is a key factor in positive therapeutic outcome. There is currently much debate about theoretical developments within the person-centred world and their application. Discussions on the theme of Rogers' therapeutic conditions presented by various key members of the person-centred community have been published (Wyatt, 2001; Haugh and Merry 2001; Bozarth and Wilkins, 2001; Wyatt and Sanders, 2002). Mearns and Thorne (2000) have produced a timely publication revising and developing key aspects of person-centred theory. Wilkins (2003) has produced a book that addresses most effectively many of the criticisms levelled against person-centred working and Embleton Tudor *et al.* (2004) give an introduction to the person-centred approach that places the theory and practice within a contemporary context.

Recently, Howard Kirschenbaum (Carl Rogers' biographer) published an article entitled 'The current status of Carl Rogers and the person-centered approach'. In his research for this article he noted that from 1946–86, 84 books, 64 chapters and 456 journal articles were published on Carl Rogers and the PCA. In contrast, from 1987–2004 there were 141 books, 174 book chapters and 462 journal articles published. These data show a clear trend towards more publications and, presumably, more readership and interest in the approach. Also, he observed that there are now 50 person-centred publications available around the world, mostly journals, and there are now person-centred organisations in 18 countries, and 20 organisations overall. He also draws attention to the large body of research demonstrating the effectiveness of person-centred therapy, concluding that the person-centred approach is 'alive and well' and appears to be experiencing 'something of a revival, both in professional activity and academic respectability' (Kirschenbaum, 2005).

There are many other books, and perhaps there is a need now for a comprehensive database of all person- or client-centred books to be made available to all training organisations and person-centred networks. (And perhaps it already exists.)

Person-centred theory affirms the importance of congruence, of being genuine, authentic, transparent; at a time when the world seems to be embracing quite the opposite. It seems to me that the relational component of the person-centred approach, based on the presence of the core conditions, is emerging strongly as a counter to the sense of isolation that frequently accompanies deep psychological and emotional problems, and which is a feature of materialistic societies. It is fascinating that this is occurring now given that the concept of relational counselling was very much a driving force in the early development of the ideas that then developed into what we know as the person-centred approach. Of the counselling relationship Rogers wrote in 1942, 'The counselling relationship is one in which warmth of acceptance and absence of any coercion or personal pressure on the part of the counsellor permits the maximum expression of feelings, attitudes, and problems by the counselee . . . In the unique experience of complete emotional freedom within a well-defined framework the client is free to recognize and understand his impulses and patterns, positive and negative, as in no other relationship' (Rogers, 1942, pp. 113–14).

This is obviously a very brief introduction to the approach and its application to working with people psychologically affected by warfare. Person-centred theory continues to develop as practitioners and theoreticians consider its application in various fields of therapeutic work and extend their theoretical understanding of developmental and therapeutic processes. At times, it feels like it has become more than just individuals, rather it feels like a group of colleagues, based around the world, working together to penetrate deeper towards a more complete theory of the human condition, and this includes people from the many traditions and schools of thought. Person- or client-centred theory and practice has a key role in this process. It is an exciting time.

PART I

Ania's story

The soldiers had come in the night . . . , Ania had tried to hide, tried to escape, but she had been seen. She was raped. They left her for dead, bleeding in the dust. Her brother lay dead, shot in the head in front of her, but only after they tortured him. They'd cut off his hands. When she was found and brought to the hospital she was barely alive herself. She was still carrying one of his hands, holding it to her heart . . . it was five days later . . .

CHAPTER I

Counselling session 1: silence and a focus on Ania's daughter, Maria

Debbie was an experienced counsellor. She had been working with people who had been victims of warfare for a few years, but she had never lost the sense of shock when she heard the stories, the horrific and tragic events that her clients brought to the counselling relationship. But it wasn't just the tales, it was the people, the way they were, the terror, the sadness, and, yes, the strength that they demonstrated in their struggle to cope. She hoped she would never lose that sense of shock. It was important for her to remain open and to be fully present, to bear the pain of being affected as a person, as a fellow human-being, when listening to others describe what had happened to them, or what they had witnessed.

She had regular supervision and she needed it. Now, she sat in the kitchen area at the counselling centre which specialised in helping people who were, and still are, the victims of war and torture. Her new client, Ania, was due any time. She had already been assessed and Debbie had seen the report. She always found it difficult knowing things about her clients before the client had told her. She didn't want to spend the first session telling the client what she knew, although she knew that would be appropriate to a spirit of openness. What she wanted was to give her client the time and the space to tell her own story, in her own way, at her own pace, something which didn't always happen in assessments. For Debbie, the process of hearing a client's story was a key element in the therapeutic process, and so she had decided some while back not to rob her clients of that by telling them what she had read. She would concentrate on building the therapeutic relationship, offering the 'core conditions', and thereby facilitate what she considered to be a healing process.

She knew that Ania had been brought over by an agency helping people affected by the war. She had refused counselling previously, not wanting to talk, simply wanting to try and make a new start. She had got a part-time job, and was making progress in her new life, but had recently started to withdraw and she had been encouraged by a support worker to seek counselling.

There was a knock at the door. 'Ania's here, Debbie.' It was Julie, the receptionist. 'Thanks, Julie.'

Debbie took a quick look around the counselling room where she now was; it was tidy, tissues and water on the table. She got up and went out to the reception area.

Ania was sitting, looking down. She looked quite thin and pale, and was holding her hands in her lap in a tense sort of way. 'Ania?'

She looked up. 'Yes.'

'Hello, I'm Debbie. Would you like to come through.'

'Yes. Thank you.'

Ania got up and followed Debbie to the counselling room.

'Please, have a seat.'

'Thank you.' Ania sat down, still wearing her coat.

Debbie wanted to keep to the non-directivenes of the person-centred approach. She was already sensing that Ania was quite withdrawn and she didn't want lengthy silences to start becoming a problem for her, or putting her off from attending. At the same time, she didn't want to come across as some well-meaning friendly face that was out of touch with the seriousness of the events in Ania's life.

'This is the first time you've been to counselling?'

Ania responded, 'yes, yes it is.'

Debbie nodded and smiled, she wanted Ania to feel welcomed and accepted. 'I don't want you to feel you have to say anything that you don't want to.'

Ania nodded.

'And there's really no rush, no pressure, and I'd really like to try and help you with what's difficult.'

Ania nodded again. She liked the thought that there would be no pressure on her to speak. She did not know what to say, and she didn't want to feel as though she was going to be made to talk about things.

'I only speak English, are you OK with the counselling being in English?'

Ania nodded. 'I learned English and it has much improved since being here. I make mistakes, but I hope you will understand.'

Debbie felt a warmth for the woman in front of her, partly because of knowing something of her background, but also because she was a person, struggling with life in her own way. 'It is not always easy to find the right words.'

'No, but I try. And I hope that you will understand.'

'I will try to and if I am not sure, is it OK if I tell you? And if there is something I say that you are not sure of, please tell me. Is that OK?'

Ania nodded and smiled.

Debbie smiled back, 'and I know we sent you information about the counselling. Did you have any questions, was there anything that you were unsure of?'

Ania shook her head.

'And that the counselling is for 50 minutes, though we can negotiate a shorter time if that is what you feel you need.'

Ania nodded. She sat and really didn't know what to say or where to begin. She hadn't spoken much about anything to anyone, and whilst she knew that she wasn't coping well, she was having terrible nightmares and feeling so low, she really had no idea what to say or how to say it. And she wasn't at all sure that she really wanted to say anything. She didn't know the woman opposite her. She seemed friendly enough, but she didn't *know* her. She needed to know her before she felt she could talk to her. She felt sure that Debbie wouldn't understand. How could she? She wouldn't have experienced what she had had to go through. How could she understand? No one could understand unless they had been through it.

Debbie sensed an awkwardness in the silence, and felt that it would be therapeutically helpful to convey her awareness of how difficult it could be to start. It also offered a reaching out to her client, and showed that she was seeking to understand the silence and how difficult it could be. 'It must be very difficult to know where to begin?'

Ania nodded but it did not take her away from her own thoughts and feelings. She felt a dark heaviness weighing her down as she continued to sit, silently staring down at the floor, but not really seeing. She was lost in her own thoughts, increasingly oblivious of the room, and of Debbie, as she sunk into those dark, heavy feelings that were all too familiar. The sounds, the noise, bombs, guns, houses, walls crashing down, screams, shouts. She closed her eyes, trying to push it away. It hadn't been like this all of the time, but recently it had all become more present. And the soldiers . . . , her brother. Her parents already dead, killed in a bombing attack. Now she was alone, except for Maria, her daughter. She loved her dearly, dearly – she was all she had. She took a deep breath and sighed. Though she didn't think of it in those terms, her psychological processes were in a sense using her love for her daughter as a barrier to the hatred and violence that had caused her to come into the world, though the memories returned in the night to stalk her and cause her to awake, sometimes screaming and always in terror.

Debbie sat silently, being with her feelings for Ania. She could only guess what Ania might be thinking. But she wasn't going to let herself drift into her own speculations. She wanted to keep her attention and focus. It was important for her to do this. She believed it to be an important feature of effective therapy. Just because there was a silence did not mean that you let your focus slip. She was there to be present, as a person, with her client. She was there to be open to whatever her client wanted to communicate, and to her own inner processes as well. She was there to experience and offer unconditional positive regard.

For Ania there was a succession of friends' faces, friends from her past, friends she had not seen now for a long while, many of whom she knew she would never see again. Most were probably dead. One day she hoped to go back, one day, but at the moment she didn't know what she wanted. She just felt trapped, trapped inside herself. And then she thought of Maria, three years old now. She felt herself smiling. How she loved her, wanted to be with her. How hard it had been to leave her when she had got a job, but the social worker had convinced her it would be OK, and it seemed to be, but she had spent the morning aching to see her again. Sweet little Maria, golden hair, blue eyes, such a happy child. And she was hers, the only thing she had in the world. She felt the darkness lifting a little as she thought of Maria and the way that she spoke. She was such a serious little girl, quite quiet in many ways, and yet she so loved to laugh and play and sing songs and dance.

They hadn't sung and danced for a few weeks now, it made Ania sad. But they still played games together and laughed, but there was a sadness in the midst of the smiles. The social worker had picked up on it when she had seen them together, and had enquired what was wrong. At first Ania had denied anything was wrong, but she had got to know and respect Gina, who was Italian, she had such a wonderful enthusiasm for life and she knew she was concerned because she also cared. She had told Gina what was happening for her and Gina had persuaded her to come for counselling.

As she sat there in the counselling room in the present, Ania had no sense of the time passing. She felt quite warm in the room, but did not want to take her coat off. She hadn't moved since they had sat down, not that she was aware of it. But Debbie was. And Debbie felt warm in the room and was sure that Ania must be uncomfortable. 'If you'd like to take your coat off . . .'

Ania didn't want to, yes, it was warm but she felt comforted by her coat. It was important to her. She'd had it for some while, actually since she had arrived in the UK. In fact, it was the first thing she had bought for herself. It was like a symbol of a new start, a new life, though she wasn't thinking in those terms as she sat, holding her coat against her.

Debbie was not going to intrude further on Ania's silence. Her two comments were genuine, and voiced out of a desire to assist. But she did not want Ania to speak because she felt she had to, or she ought to. The silence had felt awkward at first but now it felt a little easier, strangely enough, and she guessed that may be because Ania was very much in her own thoughts and maybe not so in touch with the room, with her, with the idea of being there for counselling.

Ania remained in her thoughts, still looking down. Minutes passed.

There was a crash from outside, it jolted Ania back to the room, back into the present, and she felt her heart thumping. She looked at Debbie.

'It's OK, but quite a shock, yes. I am sorry about that.'

Ania nodded. 'It is OK.'

Debbie knew that there were plenty of people around that afternoon so she didn't get up to see what had happened. She was glad of this, she didn't want to leave Ania, or give the impression that something else was more important, unless it had sounded really serious. She guessed someone had dropped something.

Debbie took the opportunity of the eye contact, and smiled slightly before speaking. 'You looked as though you were lost in thought, Ania.'

Ania nodded, she wanted to speak, she had things she needed to say, she felt her heart still thumping. She needed to start to say something, 'I . . . , yes, yes, I was thinking about so many things.'

'Mhmm, so many things to think about.'

Ania nodded, now looking towards Debbie. 'But not good things, not always.'

'No, sometimes the things that you think about are not good.'

'Bad things.' Ania dropped her eyes and looked back down towards the floor, rubbing her fingers together nervously in her lap.

'Bad things, things that have happened?'

Ania nodded again. This time, however, she made herself think about Maria, she knew she would feel easier thinking about Maria.

Debbie noticed a bit of a smile on Ania's face. 'And things that make you smile?'

Empathy is not simply about words. Body language and facial expression are also important expressive elements for the person-centred counsellor to be sensitive and responsive to. What needs to be taken into account is the fact that feelings may be conveyed through body language and facial expression that may be outside of the awareness of the client. In other words, what may be being communicated is in effect coming direct from the client's experiencing but is by-passing awareness. Primarily empathy is a response to what the client intends to communicate, but empathic responding to other communication is acceptable but there is a need to be wary where there is overmuch responding, for instance, to body language at the expense of responding to words. It can be invasive. It can cause material out of awareness to be drawn into awareness before a client is psychologically ready. A client's inner world needs to be engaged with carefully and respectfully, and not bluntly.

'I was thinking about my daughter, Maria, she's three years old. I love her so much.'

'Maria, a lovely name and you love her so much, Ania. Is it OK if I call you Ania?'

'Yes.'

'And please call me Debbie.'

'OK'

'And you were saying how much you love Maria.'

'Yes. She's all that I have, you see, she's everything to me.'

'Mhmm, everything, all you have.'

Ania was thinking about the way Maria laughed and got excited about things. 'She's got so much life, she loves people. She runs to me and hugs me. She's so good.'

'You must be very proud of her, she sounds a delightful little girl, so much life in her.'

'She likes to draw. She spends a lot of time drawing pictures of people, of places. I have so many pictures at home.'

'Mhmm.'

'She draws me a lot, I come out funny colours and shapes but she likes bright colours.'

'Mhmm, she likes to draw with bright colours, and draws you in particular.'

'And she likes to draw buildings and trees. She really concentrates, she's so, how do you say, focus?'

'Focused, she really gives everything to her drawing.'

'Yes, focused. I would like to show you some of her pictures.'

'I would love to see them.'

'I will bring some next time.' Ania felt good. She was very proud of her daughter and she wanted Debbie to see how good she was. It was important for her for people to know about Maria and to admire her.

'Thank you. I look forward to seeing them.'

'Thank you.'

A client speaks about her daughter. Presumably it is easier for her to talk about her daughter, and perhaps safer as well. However, having done so, silence returns. The counsellor stays with the silence, respecting the client's need to experience this. The topic of working with silence is an important one.

There are many forms of silence. Some silences involve a clear sense that work is in progress, others are awkward; a silence emerging out of a discomfort around what to say (and what not to), or of simply feeling something should be said but not feeling able to speak.

When a silence emerges in a session, the first response of the person-centred counsellor is to respect that silence. The most effective empathy for silence is to communicate silence back, at least until such time as something indicates a therapeutic need to speak, and then it may simply be for the counsellor to acknowledge his or her presence should the client wish to say something. Or, if there is doubt as to whether psychological contact exists, to employ a pre-therapy response along the lines of observing that '. . . is sitting in silence with . . .', using the names of the client and the counsellor.

Ania lapsed back into silence. Debbie was left with a sense of a woman whose daughter, Maria, was all-important. What had she said? "She's all I have". There was a sadness in her voice as she had said that, and yet happy, too, that she had Maria. She somehow felt that it might be a while before Ania talked about or expressed her sadness. But she accepted that it could take time, this was the first session and if the therapeutic relationship was to develop around Ania's feelings towards her daughter, that was fine. She, Debbie, could accept that.

In the past Debbie would have been trying to strike up conversation with clients. She had found it hard to stay with a silence, always wanting to fill it, and generally, she eventually understood, because she was needing to for her own sense of ease. Now, unless a client seemed particularly disturbed by long silences, she would allow them to continue, occasionally reminding her client of her presence and that she was there for them.

Debbie was thinking about what Ania had said, about the 'bad things' she had been thinking about. She knew she was experiencing an urge to ask what they were, but at the same time she knew she should let Ania tell her when she wanted to.

'It can be so difficult to talk about things, particularly "bad things", and some-times we don't want to, sometimes we'd rather talk about nice things, and sometimes we just don't know what we want to say. We just don't know where to begin.' Debbie spoke from a sense of Ania's ability to talk about the nice things like Maria, but could only make reference to "bad things" with saying anything more.

Ania sat tight-lipped. She knew she wanted to speak, but she was afraid of speak-ing, afraid that if she started she might not stop, that if she spoke about what she knew she felt inside, she might lose control, feel worse, not be able to cope. She felt like she had to . . . . She sighed.

'A big sigh.'

'I think I am a bit afraid.'

'Afraid? Can you tell me what is making you afraid?'

It is not unusual for a client to fear that if they begin to talk and to express feelings and emotion, they may never stop, that they will be completely overwhelmed within the experience to the degree that they will feel unable to contain, cope with or even survive the process. Calm reassurance from the counsellor and acknowledgement of those fears where they are being communicated, are important, conveyed with the warm acceptance that is expressive of the counsellor's unconditional positive regard.

'There is so much to tell but I am not sure that I can tell it without making myself worse.'

'You are afraid that if you tell me about the bad things it will just make you feel worse?'

'I am sure it will.'

'It can be painful, yes, and sometimes it is helpful to talk to someone and to be listened to.'

'I don't think you will understand.'

'I may not, but I will be trying to understand, and if it is something I do not under-stand, may I ask you?'

'Yes, that would be good.'

'Thank you.'

Ania thought for a moment. 'I want to tell you about my country.'

'I would like to hear about your country, Ania.'

Whilst this response is not empathic to what the client has said, it is perhaps empathic to a sensed need in the client to know that the counsellor wants to hear her story. The counsellor's response is genuine and authentic. A person-centred counsellor would not, of course, say they wanted to hear the story if they were feeling bored with what the client was saying. They would take their reaction to supervision.

In an established therapeutic relationship there may also be times when the counsellor would share their reaction as it could have therapeutic value. For example, a client keeps repeating the same story over and over again, and it is likely they do that with lots of people and are wondering why no one wants to spend time with them. However, if the counsellor felt a "bored not wanting to listen reaction" in this situation between Ania and Debbie, then it would very definitely not be disclosed and would need to be addressed in supervision at the earliest opportunity.

'Then I will tell you, Deb-bie.' It was the first time that Ania had said "Debbie" and it felt good to have said it. It was a new name to her, she had not heard it before.

Ania spoke of her country before the war, of the fields and the towns, of where she played as a child. She did not speak of her parents, or her brother, but of herself and of places. Debbie respected what Ania was choosing to talk about, and not talk about. 'So you have lots of memories of your childhood, Ania?'

Ania nodded. 'It was good. We enjoyed ourselves.'

Debbie noticed the first use of we.

'You enjoyed yourselves – it is good to have those memories.'

Ania then began to talk about her father and mother. It seemed that under the communist system her family were quite well off, her father worked for the government, something to do with the communist party, and was very well respected. Her mother worked in a factory. It seems that they were very happy, and that she had lots of friends. Although her country then was the former Yugoslavia, her family was in fact Croatian. They lived in Bosnia.

Time passed and the session was due to end. Debbie pointed out the time and Ania stopped speaking.

'Would you like to come again next week and maybe bring some of Maria's drawings?'

'Yes, I will ask her which ones she would like me to bring.'

'That would be nice.'

Ania left, feeling good about what she had said. She had begun to like Debbie. She seemed really interested and she did listen. She had asked a couple of times about things she did not understand and that felt good for Ania, it made her believe even more that Debbie wanted to understand. Ania headed back home and got ready to go and collect Maria from the childminder that Gina had arranged so she could come to the counselling. She was looking forward to seeing Maria. They had only been apart for a couple of hours, but that was too long for Ania, they generally spent the afternoons together.

Points for discussion

- How would you have introduced yourself to Ania? What would you have felt it important to communicate at the start?
- How would you have handled the silence? Evaluate how Debbie dealt with it.

- What are your impressions of Ania and what image does she give to you?
- What evidence of person-centred practice did you notice in the session? Please be specific.
- Would you be experiencing any particular concerns from that session? Do you have any expectations as to the nature of future sessions?
- Write notes for this session.

CHAPTER 2

Issues of confidentiality

Debbie was sitting at the Counselling Centre when the phone rang. It was Julie, the receptionist. 'I have a call for you, it's Gina, social worker for one of your clients, wants to have a word.'

'Sure, no problem.'

Debbie immediately realised that she hadn't checked whether she had her client's permission to talk to her social worker. She didn't feel able to say much, but she appreciated that social services may well be monitoring to ensure Maria's well-being. Maybe there was a problem, she couldn't get to the session later that day. She took a moment and just thought it through before saying to Julie, 'OK, put her through.'

'Hello, Debbie speaking, can I help?'

'Hello, yes, this is Gina, Ania's social worker.'

'Hello Gina. How can I help?'

'Well, I wanted to check that all was OK with Ania. I know that you probably can't say much because of confidentiality, but we are, of course, concerned and wanting to make sure that Maria is OK. I really wanted to touch base and see how things are.'

'Yes, I haven't discussed talking with you, but, yes, Ania has attended her first appointment and is due to come again today. It's early days, of course. Can you tell me if you have particular concerns?'

'We don't really have any, and I don't want to intrude on confidentiality, it's just that I was wondering if she has said much about her past. We're hoping that she will. We think she's been containing a lot of feelings, memories and traumas.'

'I am sure that's very likely. I don't take a history, rather give my clients time to tell their story as they wish and as they feel able. Does she talk about it much with you?'

'No, we don't go into that, more concerned with how she is with Maria.'

'Have you concerns about that?'

'No, we are very pleased. She seems to be a very happy little girl.'

'Good.'

'It would be good to be aware what progress she is making. As you may know, there are issues around trafficking and, well, we are sure Ania and Maria came over with a reputable agency, but you cannot be sure. Traffickers can come back, particularly where the mother is expecting a child, to look for the child. And for young women as well. It's a real problem. We have to have this in mind, particularly if there are any signs of anxiety in Ania towards Maria's safety. Can we keep in touch?'

'Sure and I will talk to Ania about "progress reports". As you probably know, we do hold a very clear boundary of confidentiality here, particularly given the difficult experiences many of our clients have. They often do need very clear assurances that what they say will be kept confidential. And I am aware of the difficulty where there are childcare issues, and of course, if there is concern about anything like you have suggested then we will get in touch. Yes, I am aware of the problem. There are so many complexities in these situations.'

'Yes, very much so, and, well, you've probably witnessed mothers with real mixed feelings towards a child that was conceived through rape.'

'Yes. Yes, I wonder what might be present for Ania, as with any mother in this situation, that she may be denying to her awareness. She certainly speaks lovingly of Maria.'

'And we see that as well. Yes, she is very loving. We just need to monitor the situation.'

'Sure.'

The conversation drew to a close and Debbie put the phone down and made a mental note to talk to Ania about Gina wanting progress reports. She also noted that she would mention this to the manager at the centre. This situation did arise and the response was generally to agree to maintain confidentiality unless there were concerns for Maria's well-being, and even then it would necessitate a discussion (which would include the client) on a course of action. It was a difficult area requiring great sensitivity from everyone.

The question of sharing information with other professionals working with a client is often an area in need of clarification. Not all professionals understand the meaning that counsellors ascribe to confidentiality. Equally, counsellors often do not appreciate that different professionals have different meanings to confidentiality. In a GP surgery, or a community mental health team, for example, confidentiality may be boundaried within the multi-disciplinary team, not just to one individual. But with counselling the confidentiality contract is clear – between the client and the counsellor unless certain disclosures are made that will require the counsellor to breach confidentiality which may be a statutory or legal requirement, or explicit to the contractual arrangements made between an employer and the counsellor – for instance, a school requiring disclosure of drug use to be passed on to the headperson.

Counsellors can be perceived as 'precious' when it comes to confidentiality. It is important not to encourage this view, rather to explain the meaning that counsellor's ascribe to confidentiality. There is still a lot of education needed to ensure that other professionals appreciate the nature of counselling.

In the situation with Ania and Debbie, Gina is asking about progress reports and highlighting the relationship between Ania and Maria, presumably concerned should there be childcare issues. This is a reasonable concern, though Gina is indicating that they are happy with Ania and Maria. Were Debbie to be concerned about Ania's parenting and behaviour towards Maria, suspecting that Maria was being harmed or at risk of being harmed, then this should be discussed with the client and in supervision, and if it needs to go further, with the manager of the agency. All agencies that employ counsellors – paid or voluntary – should have a policy and a protocol on responding to situations where breaching confidentiality is to be considered. But there is also a need for flexibility to take into account the uniqueness of each situation given the individual experiencing and behaviour of each person involved.

The notion of progress reports would have to be agreed between all parties, and what they would contain. It is likely that the person-centred counsellor would not want to pass on any information that has not been agreed by the client. In general, in my experience, unless there are specific and serious issues of concern such as child protection issues, progress reports are more likely to take the form of confirming attendance, and may occasionally include mention of issues being addressed but without unnecessary detail.

Within all of the above, the person-centred counsellor will seek to maintain the value and attitudes of the person-centred approach. It is not an easy area.

Counselling session 2: sadness and anger at the death of her parents

Ania arrived promptly and Debbie had gone out to meet her in the reception area. They returned to the counselling room.

'Can I take your coat?'

'Yes please, thank you.'

Debbie took Ania's coat and hung it on the back of the door. She noticed that she had a folder in her bag that she was getting out as she put it down.

'The drawings?'

'Yes, and I would like you to see them.'

Debbie decided not to cut across Ania's intention to show her the drawings straight away by bringing up her conversation with Gina. But she intended to mention it at the earliest opportunity when it would hopefully not disrupt the therapeutic process.

'OK, where do you want to start?'

'I told Maria that Mama was spending time talking to a nice woman called Debbie, and that she was interested in her drawings. And I said that she should choose which ones I would bring. She gave it a lot of thought but eventually she decided on these.' Ania proceeded to take them out of the folder. 'This is the first one, she wanted you to see this first, it is a picture of Maria and me going shopping. See, she has drawn a red shopping bag.'

'Yes I do. And what a lot of yellow hair she has drawn.'

'Yes, she has a lot of hair, it is not yellow, but that is the closest colour that she had.'

'And you are both smiling?'

'Yes, we like to go shopping together.'

'Wonderful.'

Ania was passing over the next picture. 'This is a picture of our garden. It is a small garden, but it has a tree and a fence, as you can see. And this is Maria running around with a ball.'

Debbie looked at the picture closely. It really was quite good. Bright colours, yes, but drawn not too hard. The tree was a brown pole with a mass of green on it, and what she guessed must be a little brown bird sitting on it.

'A bird?' Debbie enquired.

'Yes. She likes birds. We feed the pigeons in the park. She has a picture of that here.' Ania looked through the drawings. 'Yes, here we are.' She handed it to Debbie.

'Thank you.' Debbie smiled, 'What a lot of pigeons! Little dark shapes with little heads, and some with wings, dotted all over the picture.'

'Yes.'

Ania passed another picture across to Debbie. 'And this is our house. We live downstairs. She has coloured in the door and the curtains, and that is Maria at the window here, and me at that window there.'

'And she spends a lot of time drawing and colouring?'

'It is what she spends a lot of time doing. She really likes it.'

Ania showed Debbie the rest of the pictures. She had brought ten in all. In a way it was a bit like someone coming and showing you their photos except that it wasn't, it was much more personal, there was so much feeling in Ania attached to the pictures that Maria had drawn. Debbie could imagine Ania covering the walls with them.

After she had seen them all, Debbie said, 'I think they are lovely. Please thank Maria for letting me see them.'

'She wants you to have one of them.'

'Are you sure?'

'Yes, she was very sure.'

'Which one? I like them all.'

'She wanted you to have this one, of our house with us at the windows.'

'Well thank you very much, and please thank Maria for me. I will put it on my wall at home. Would Maria like me to put it there, do you think?'

'Yes.'

'Well, I am very pleased. It's a lovely drawing. She's a very talented little girl.'

'I will tell her. She will be pleased that you like them.'

'And you must be very pleased with them as well?'

'I am.' Ania suddenly seemed to change, her expression suddenly lost its shine that had been there whilst she had enthused about Maria's pictures.

'What's wrong, Ania?' Debbie spoke softly, the concern in her voice congruently matching the concern that she was feeling. The change had been sudden and dramatic.

> The counsellor empathises with the client's facial expression and the experienced change in the relational atmosphere. However, rather than the somewhat directive question, 'what's wrong?', she could have simply acknowledged her experience, for example, 'you look concerned, Ania, and I am aware that something suddenly feels different.'

'It's OK. It is nothing.'

'Nothing?'

> Is the counsellor, with her questioning tone, now encouraging directive-ness? Is she directing Ania into an area of her experiencing that she simply may not want or feel ready to share? Have Debbie's responses encouraged Ania to feel pressure to disclose? Is she being facilitative or directive? The person-centred counsellor will seek to be facilitative. The client may only disclose because of the pressure. Of course, she may have disclosed whatever the response from Debbie, but even then there will remain the matter as to how the client will have interpreted and experienced Debbie's words. She might be left feeling that is someone who is going to probe into sensitive areas. That could cause the client to defend against this, and the most powerful defence is to stop attending.
>
> There is a need for great sensitivity as the counsellor seeks to be the companion to the client on their journey, letting the client choose the path, and not to be the leader encouraging them to travel in a particular direction or by a particular route.

Ania could feel such deep sadness within her. It was a familiar feeling and one she sought to keep from the view of others. It was one that she shared with the dark night when Maria was fast asleep, often the result of something joyful Ania had done during the day, and there was no one there to share it with. Suddenly it seemed as though the feelings were threatening to engulf her. Her stomach was tight, and she swallowed as she fought back the tears.

'It's safe to let it go.' Debbie spoke softly, seeking to reassure her. Ania heard her voice but she didn't want to, she was scared, terrified of how it would be, how she would be. She remembered that awful thud, and the dust, the shouts, people running, looking out at the scene where there should have been a wall. Half of the house had gone, just rubble. They were gone, gone in one awful moment. She swallowed again, and sniffed, reaching over for a tissue.

Debbie watched her, she could see the pain and grief that was wracking Ania's thin body. She could only imagine what awful feelings were present, the heartache and the loss. She knew the facts from the assessments, but that wasn't the human tragedy, that didn't capture the pain and horror that was perhaps now being re-lived before her.

Ania's breath was coming in short, sharp intakes, and swallows, she opened her mouth as if to speak but the words seemed to be snatched back into her throat.

'Take your time Ania, try and breathe slowly if you can.'

Her breathing was still in short and sharp breaths, she shook her head, unable to say or do anything.

Debbie reached over and held her hand, trying to offer warmth and reassurance at a time when she could only imagine how little reassurance and warmth was probably present within Ania's life.

The counsellor seeks to convey genuine and authentic warm acceptance of her client. Her response comes from the heart. Yes, Debbie is in the relationship as a counsellor, but she uses her self – we should say is being herself. Part of being a human-being is having a heart. Debbie's response is heartfelt. It is a spontaneous act arising out of the therapeutic relationship and the communication that is passing between the client and the counsellor.

Ania was grateful for the contact. She didn't have much physical contact with people these days, except with Maria. It felt good feeling Debbie's warm hands holding her. 'I . . . , oh God . . . , I . . . , I'm . . .'. Still the breaths came short, sharp, after each one Ania closed her mouth before letting the air out, and then another short breath. She swallowed again. 'They . . . , were . . . , just . . . , just . . . ', the breathing stopped her speaking again.

'They were just . . . ?' Debbie gently squeezed Ania's hand as she spoke, seeking to convey reassurance.

Ania looked at Debbie. 'I wish . . . ,' she swallowed, ' . . . I so wish they had known Maria.' Ania closed her eyes and her body began to convulse with the sobs. The tears streamed down her face.

Debbie took a deep breath herself and increased the pressure on Ania's hand. Ania brought her other hand across and held on tightly.

'They never knew her, they died before any of it happened.' She swallowed again, opened her eyes and reached for a tissue. 'I miss them so much.'

Debbie guessed that she was talking about her parents having read the assessment that had outlined that they had died during some kind of a bomb attack. 'They were your parents . . . '

There is an assumption being made, although it is informed. It proves facilitative as it is a reasonable assumption to make, but it robs Ania of saying, in
her own words, and with her own feelings expressed through those words,
that it is her parents that she is referring to. It might have been more facilitative to have responded with a simply empathic statement, 'you so wish
they had known Maria'.

Ania nodded. 'I can see their faces so clearly still from that last day, having
dinner.' She paused and closed her eyes. 'We had eaten dinner and they were
sitting in the lounge together, listening to the radio, I think. I don't know. I was
in my room.' Another pause. 'There were explosions. Everything shook, and
then ...' Ania re-lived the explosion that had taken her parents away from
her and destroyed a large section of the house. She felt herself shaking. Debbie
noticed that her colour had paled. Ania was still with the images, the memories. The wall had disappeared. '... there was dust everywhere and I could
see out. I was confused, I didn't understand. Then I remember screaming,
"mama, papa", but the rest of the house had gone. Neighbours were running,
they tried to find them, but it was too late. They had no chance. The ambulance
arrived, they took me to the hospital. I don't remember much. I had cuts and
bruises. They found my parents but they were both dead.' She could see their
bodies after they had been laid out. They'd cleaned them up as best they could,
but their bodies were broken.
'I remember crying when I saw them and feeling so angry. They'd been taken
from me by those bastard Serbs. I wanted to kill them, kill them all. They had
no right to do that. They are murderers, all of them.'
Debbie sat close to Ania, still holding her hand. 'So much for you to feel angry
about, wanting to kill, wanting revenge.'

Debbie has not empathised with what Ania has said – perhaps she feels a
reluctance to blame the Serbs? There is a need for self-questioning as
to why it was a partial empathic response. The person-centred counsellor
will want to hear and be able to convey that they have heard all that has
been said.

Ania remembered her brother coming home, but she couldn't think of her brother,
not now, the image of him tortured and dying forced itself into her mind. It was
too overwhelming, she couldn't talk about her brother. But it added to her
anger. Her jaw had tightened, her eyes suddenly blazing and intense.
'I would like to kill many Serbs, they did terrible things and they must be punished. I would cut them, kill them, shoot them, stamp on their faces and crush
their bones. They do not deserve to live.'

'Hate them, want to cut them, kill them, shoot them, stamp on their faces and crush their bones.' Debbie spoke with more intensity, reflecting Ania's tone of voice.

> This is much clearer empathy, strengthened by the mirroring of the voice tone.

'So many people suffered, so many people ...' Ania's voice trailed off. She suddenly felt drained, exhausted. The tears, the emotional release had taken its toll.

Debbie nodded. 'I cannot begin to understand what it was like, but I can sense the hurt, the pain, the anguish, the anger that you are feeling.' She paused momentarily, picking up on what Ania had just said. 'So much suffering, so many people, so many people ...'

'And here I am in England, trying to make a new life. I, who have seen and felt so much, so many bad things, and trying to give Maria a home and a life.' She looked at Debbie. 'She keeps me alive.'

Debbie nodded, her own heart reaching out to Ania. She felt there was no need for words, she believed that the look in her eyes would convey her feelings.

Ania saw the compassion, and somehow it was comforting. 'Thank you.'

> Once more, it is not through words that warm acceptance, unconditional positive regard and empathy for what the client is experiencing is being conveyed. The counsellor should never underestimate the communicative power of eye contact. The person-centred counsellor well appreciates that they need to bring their whole selves into the counselling relationship, including their physical responses to what is being said and felt.
>
> The self-development work that the counsellor has undertaken will ensure that there is a greater likelihood of congruence between their thoughts, feelings and body language, ensuring that the client receives a consistent response and not a mixed message which can confuse and undermine trust, and the therapeutic nature of the relationship.

'I can only offer you myself, my being here with you, as a human-being, as a woman, as a mother.' Debbie hadn't planned to say "as a mother", but it was true. She was there as herself, as the various identities that made up who she was. And she was a counsellor, but she knew that in this moment, at this time, she was not there as a counsellor. It wasn't being a counsellor that could stand or sit beside a person in such pain and communicate some kind of human solidarity. It was by being a human-being, touched and affected by what she was witnessing, hearing, experiencing, being open and prepared to communicate what was present in her awareness.

The two women sat for a while in silence. Debbie had noticed that time was moving on and the session would need to end soon. She mentioned this, and Ania nodded, and gradually withdrew from the contact.

'It's been a hard session for you, Ania, for both of us, but for you especially. Take care of yourself after you leave. You may feel a little disorientated after the release of so much feeling, and connecting with memories in such a powerful way.'

Ania nodded. 'This is what counselling means, does it not?'

'Yes, it can be this way.'

'Yes. I expected it would be. It is difficult but necessary, yes?'

Debbie nodded.

'I must keep coming.'

'And I will be here for as long as it takes.'

'Thank you, Debbie.'

Debbie remembered Gina. 'Oh, I nearly forgot, Gina called, wanting to know how you were progressing.'

'Yes, she is very concerned.'

'We don't usually give out information, not unless you give us permission, and then only basic information, not all the details of what you say or what happens.'

'I understand. I am happy with you speaking to Gina. She is good to me.'

'Then if she calls I will say that you are working through the difficulties and you want to continue. But I will not be specific. She has said you do not speak of these things to her and, well, I want to respect that and not communicate anything that you have chosen not to say.'

Ania was a little surprised, but it also felt good. There were things she had chosen not to discuss with Gina. She might do in the future, she didn't know. But she was happy for her not to know. Gina could ask lots of questions and she did not always want to answer them. And there were things she did not want to be asked about.

'Yes. That is acceptable to me.'

'She asked about progress reports as well. We don't usually write reports like that, but I can keep her updated on the phone, but I don't want her to get too involved in the counselling work. That's why I don't want to go into a lot of detail.'

'OK.'

Debbie nodded. 'Good. I needed to mention it.'

'That is OK.' Ania smiled.

'Thank Maria for the picture.'

'I will.' Ania was getting up and Debbie was reaching for her coat. 'I will see you next week, yes?'

'Yes, at the same time.'

'That is good. Until then.' Ania put out her hand, and Debbie took it. She was struck how formal Ania sounded. Perhaps it was partly her grasp of English, but she sensed as well that it was something about her preparing herself to go back out into the world, back out on her own to try and contain the feelings and the memories that must trouble her so. She watched Ania leave and sat back down to reflect on the session and to write her notes.

Points for discussion

- How would you have handled the call from the social worker? Assess Debbie's handling of the situation.
- How did Debbie convey unconditional positive regard in this session? What effect did it have? Be specific.
- What significant therapeutic moments did you identify within the session?
- How did you respond to Debbie's comments towards the end of the session regarding communication with Gina? How might it have been handled differently?
- Do you feel Debbie was inappropriate in any of her responses and, if so, why? How might she have responded differently?
- What issues do you feel Debbie could usefully take to supervision from this session?
- Write notes for this session.

CHAPTER 3

Counselling session 3: client cancels as her daughter is unwell

There was a phone call for Debbie who had just arrived at the centre.

'Hello, Debbie?'

'Yes, hello Ania. How are you?'

'Maria is not well today and I will need to stay and look after her. I am sorry.'

'That's OK, Ania, I hope it is nothing serious.'

'I don't think it is serious. She has an ear infection and a high temperature. So I need to stay with her.'

'OK. I hope she is soon feeling better.'

'I do too.' There was a pause and the sound of crying in the background. 'I must go now. Maria is crying.'

'Yes, I hear her. I hope she is soon feeling better. And I will see you next week at the same time, yes?'

'Yes, I will see you then. Thank you, Debbie.'

'That's OK. See you next week. Bye bye.'

'Bye bye.'

Debbie put the phone down and shook her head slightly as she thought about Ania's situation. In a foreign country, three year old daughter unwell, going through counselling to try to resolve traumas from her past, no doubt knowing she needs Maria to be better so that she can go back to work – yes, she did have enormous respect for Ania. She hoped that the counselling would help her. She knew it could never take away the past, but talking it out, releasing emotions, sharing it with another person who was offering the core conditions, she knew that it helped people to move on in themselves. Not that Ania would ever forget the past, but it was as though people who experience severe trauma become locked into that traumatic experience and then find it difficult to break free. She could imagine that Ania would have found a way initially to block it out, using Maria. But now the feelings and memories were pushing back and hence her mood had come down, and Debbie knew instinctively that it was likely to get worse before there might be some ease for Ania. She would need to re-integrate the parts of her that carried the pain and hurt, and find her own way – was that the right way of describing it? Maybe it was more about developing a way of being, a way of perceiving and experiencing her life, and herself, so that she could in some way find some kind of acceptance? No, that didn't sound or feel quite right either.

The words felt cumbersome, and Debbie didn't really feel they captured what Ania faced. In fact, the more she pondered on it, the more she began to realise she didn't have words for Ania's process. She did not know what the outcome of the counselling would be. All she could hope for was that Ania would have the strength to cope with her losses in her life, with the traumatic events that she had witnessed and been a part of. But she knew that within Ania was an actualising tendency, a fundamental urge towards making the best of things, to grow and develop. Maybe it was about finding resilience that was already present. Perhaps it was just that at times it was so much harder, yet the resilience remained and she felt sure that it could become a focus for the actualising tendency as Ania experienced the core conditions. But she knew it was speculation, and may not be how things would work out, or how they needed to be for Ania at this time.

Debbie was very aware of how much Ania was coping by doing things for Maria. That was her focus. She was not yet in a position, it seemed, to do anything for herself. It seemed that she put herself second to Maria, which was natural and yet it felt more intense, more dependent in some way. She acknowledged that she hoped that this would change in time, but for the moment Maria was the centre of Ania's life and her motivation to keep on going, and as a mother herself she could only imagine how Ania must feel when Maria was unwell, yet with a sense that it would be even more intense, perhaps.

Supervision session 1: the counsellor has knowledge that the client has not disclosed

'You work with so many people who are badly affected by trauma, Debbie, I really respect your strength, your compassion, your dedication to the work at the centre.'

'Thanks, Rob, part of me wants to react by saying "oh, it's nothing", but I know that it isn't nothing. Yes, it is hard, but I wouldn't want to be anywhere else.'

'You seem to have a natural empathy towards your clients. You seem to be able to stand or should I say sit beside them and be strong.'

'I suppose I tune in. I don't know why. Ever since working there it has felt like home, somehow. Working with people affected by war, it feels like if you are going to offer counselling, and really extend yourself, really bring healing into a place of greatest need – well, that's it. What my clients have faced – torture, rape, witnessed acts of unspeakable violence, losing their families, homes, country, everything – it brings you, it brings me, right down to a sort of bottom line.'

'A bottom line?'

'There are no techniques in that place, nothing I can do to make a difference, Rob. It's not about doing. These, my clients, are human-beings, traumatised by events. Their faith, belief, in human-beings probably undermined. They *know* what people are capable of doing to each other. They have experienced it, witnessed it, been the victim of it. They are in another place to most people.'

Rob nodded, noting the passion and the emotion in Debbie's voice. 'Hmm. That knowing . . .'

'Yes, it is that knowing. We can see things on TV, read about it in the newspapers, and, yes, we can be affected, and we are. But it is distant from our reality. We have not experienced the terror, the utter terror, of living somewhere where we are at risk of being taken and tortured, or killed. And yes, people in those places do get on with their lives, they find ways of coping in spite of these possibilities, but what they feel, what they know, what they have experienced, becomes locked inside them. People take actions that they know will put themselves at risk as well, standing up against governments where they know that they could be taken and killed or tortured. These people are heroes, absolute heroes. And they probably won't think of themselves like that, they are doing what they believe to be right, often out of a sense of utter despair, or a total conviction that they need to follow a particular course of action to try to bring about change.' Debbie stopped and sighed.

'Yes, your clients put life in perspective, somehow. I wonder if it leaves you less tolerant of people with minor problems?'

Debbie nodded and smiled. 'Only those who keep whining about them.' Debbie paused, acknowledging to herself the truth of what Rob had just said. It was a danger. She did notice that tendency in herself though she felt clear that she did not bring that into her counselling relationships. 'Yes, it probably does leave me feeling somewhat more intolerant. It makes me angry, Rob, at the injustice in our world, at the failure – time and time again – of governments to intervene to stop human tragedies, to stop genocide, to . . . Oh, I don't know. I see so many people, scarred and wounded, and I don't mean an emotional bruise here or a psychological cut there, people who are emotionally and physically beaten down, and yet they are getting on with their lives. And it is that more than anything else that motivates me, I think, the human spirit, the power of the human spirit to survive, to keep going, to find ways of continuing however much has been lost or damaged.' She shook her head as she looked towards Rob. 'It's people, Rob; people, wanting to live, wanting to rebuild their shattered lives, wanting the same things that we all want – people to love and to be loved by, security, warmth, a bit of independence.'

'I think you are right, Debbie. We do not emphasise enough the urge to live, the will to exist, if you like, that is so formidable within people. Perhaps with this client group we are brought closest to that, we see it in its raw form, and perhaps there is something about this that is inspiring to us.'

Debbie had not thought of it quite like that before, the idea of a raw will to live, but it made sense as she thought about it. 'Maybe you are right. It makes me think that there is something about my clients that tells me they have reasons enough to give up, but they don't. And perhaps it is in this that something

important exists. It's like I have a . . . , yes, it's like I have a fundamental acceptance that they could give up and it would be quite acceptable . . . , yes, I have
an acceptance of the possibility of their giving up, it's like the relationship has
a reality to it. But in a different way, somehow. It's really hard to explain what
I mean.'

'Different to working with other client groups?'

'Yes, and yet I also want to qualify that because people can find so many different
difficulties too much to bear or cope with.' Debbie paused. 'I think it's because I
am more accepting of the likelihood that people will, or could, give up, but they
don't. And you know, I sometimes wonder if that is a cultural thing, or simply a
human reaction to adversity, real adversity, where a person has looked over
the edge, faced death, faced the horrors of life, and survived. Maybe that raw,
will to live that you describe is something for us all to discover, but there must
be ways other than to face the horrors of war and trauma.' Debbie's thoughts
were with Ania. 'I need to talk about a new client, Rob, who I've seen twice.
Her name is Ania, she is Croatian but lived in Bosnia. Her parents were killed
by a bomb hitting her house, she survived. She hasn't told me all of the details,
but I have seen the assessment sheet, and I have to say that increasingly I am
realising that I do not want to have this information before I start to work with
a client, and I think I must say something.'

Where another person has been required to provide an initial assessment
session the issue arises as to what the counsellor should or needs to be
made aware of – if anything. If the assessment is to ensure a client is appropriate for counselling (and this raises the further issue of who decides that
from a person-centred theoretical viewpoint that the client is an expert on
their difficulties) then information does not need to be passed on to the counsellor. The difficulty is that because other theoretical approaches aim to
'treat' specific 'conditions' that have been 'diagnosed', the approach of the
person-centred counsellor may not be understood or valued.

The counsellor does not need to know what is to be treated, they are not
treating a condition, but accepting their client as persons and inviting them
into a therapeutic experience. Through that process, healing may occur,
growth may occur, change may occur, or the person may choose to remain
as they are. Whatever the outcome, it is likely that the client will experience
feeling empowered to make their own choices, or where this feels impossible,
to have a deeper understanding of themselves and be more completely in
contact with themselves and the more likely to engage in authentic living
which, arguably, is the goal of therapy, if there is to be an ownership of a
goal from a person-centred perspective.

'Having information from the assessment is affecting the therapeutic process?'

'It means I know what a client has experienced before they have told me. And,
yes, I could tell them right at the start, and sometimes I do, but I didn't with

Ania. I really felt that I needed to let her tell me, at her own pace, in her own time, and when she wanted me to know, when she wanted to trust me. But I'm left now knowing what she does not know I know.'

'Are you sure? Are you making an assumption here?'

'How do you mean?'

'She has been assessed. She has said things. Don't you think she naturally assumes that the information will be passed on to you?'

'I really hadn't thought of it quite like that. Well, I suppose I had, but somehow not with Ania. And I don't know why.'

'So you have thought differently towards Ania?'

'It's like, yes, I have. I haven't made clear what I know, and I have assumed, and probably falsely, that she thinks I am not aware of information about her life that she has not told me.'

'You have no reason to think that.'

'No, I don't, so something is happening here, something about Ania.'

'Mhmm, or about her story.'

Debbie took a deep breath. 'Yes. Yes.' She brought her hands up to her face. 'I can tell you what Ania has told me so far, and process that, or I can tell you what I know, and process that.'

'Which do you want to focus on?' Rob trusted Debbie to know what she needed to focus on, though his sense was that she probably needed to focus on what she knew as that seemed to have affected her and how she was relating to Ania.

'It's what I know, isn't it?'

'I think so too. You hold information about Ania that you are keeping secret.'

'And so is she. What I am keeping from her, she is keeping from me as well.'

'Mhmm.'

'It doesn't feel good, but to tell her what I know would be to direct her towards something that she may not be ready to tell me.'

'Mhmm.'

'So I can't tell her, can I?'

'No.'

'But I . . . , so what do I do?'

'What do you need to do?'

'Not let what I know affect how I am with her.'

'So, you have to not let what you know about Ania's life affect how you interact with her.'

'But I won't be transparent.'

'Do you have to be transparent about everything?'

'No, but this is about my client, surely I have to be transparent about everything related to her?'

'So, ''surely we have to be transparent about everything that we are aware of that relates to our clients?'' Is that right?'

Debbie was frowning. 'I need to be congruently present in the relationship. I need to be open to, and aware of, my own experiencing, and be able to communicate what I am experiencing to my client.'

'Do you communicate everything that you are experiencing to your clients?'

'No, no, of course not. No, that's pseudo-congruence, or false congruence, just saying things because you experience them without any thought of appropriateness or relevance.'

Congruence is not *transparency* to the point that the counsellor says anything they think or feel, justifying it because the urge came to them whilst they were with a client. Person-centred counselling does have a discipline to it, others might prefer to consider it in terms of having clear boundaries as to what is acceptable.

Congruence does not justify endless self-disclosure. Anything the counsellor says that is not empathic has to express unconditional positive regard or communicate something that is therapeutically justifiable. If in doubt, don't disclose, and take it to supervision.

This might be a cause for debate but a client is less likely to be damaged by something helpful not being said than by something unhelpful being said.

'Or our own motivation for disclosure.'

'Yes.'

'So we don't communicate experiences simply because we are aware of them, yes?'

'Mhmm. Yes. I can see where this is leading. I am aware of experiencing knowledge about Ania. But it is whether my being aware of it means I have to communicate it. OK, so what are my reasons for choosing to share something that I am experiencing? It has relevance to what is happening in that moment with a client, it is something that emerges as a result of the therapeutic relationship and persists, it is something that becomes so present that it obstructs or obscures the clarity and accuracy of my empathy.'

'Hmm.' Rob did not make further comment, he wanted to allow Debbie to follow her own process and reach her own conclusion.

Debbie paused and reflected on what she had just said. 'Well, it has relevance … Or does it? If it is not what Ania is talking about, if she is not focusing on that experience in her life with me, then, does it have relevance in that moment? I guess not.'

'OK.'

'Is it something that has emerged as a result of our relationship, well, no, it's something I had before we even met, so it hasn't emerged, it isn't some particular insight or reaction that has taken shape because of what is happening between us.'

'Right.'

'Does it obscure my empathy? I don't think so. I know what I know. I'm not finding myself dwelling on it in the session, though, well, not to that extent.'

'Hmm. So, where does that leave you?'

'I say nothing.'

Rob nodded. 'You say nothing. What will it achieve now by saying it?'

'It'll cut across Ania's process.'

Rob nodded. 'Sometimes we have to hold what we know. We are aware of it, we are holding it in awareness, but choosing not to voice it for therapeutic reasons. That feels acceptable to me, particularly in this context, maybe not in other contexts, but I am not thinking of that at this moment.'

Debbie was struck by a thought. 'Of course, it might be something that becomes more present for me.'

'Yes, and it is likely to be felt that way perhaps as Ania gets closer to disclosing to you what you already know.'

'As though the "secret" is coming into emergence.'

'And you both sense that pressure of emergence, if you like. But it is Ania's process that matters, we are, of course, "client-centred" in our practice. Her process is paramount, yes?'

Debbie nodded. 'I have supervision to sort my process out!'

'Yes. That is part of our professionalism, and what enables us to be personally present with our clients. Supervision helps us to balance the personal and the professional, yes?'

'Isn't that what it is about? Enabling us to be personally and professionally present with our clients, enabling us to ensure that anything that is affecting our ability to offer the core conditions to them is addressed and resolved?'

'Personal and the professional, that would make a good book title! I think it captures something.'

'For me working with my clients, the personal is so important.'

'Hmm. Particularly important?'

Debbie nodded. 'Yes. I have a real sense that all I have to offer is me, myself, who I am, a person, a woman, a human-being. I have nothing in a toolkit to resolve things, make things better. I have myself and I have a real sense with my clients, and particularly when addressing really traumatic incidents, and the intense emotions and hurt that are associated, that I stand naked, psychologically speaking.'

'Hmm, I hear that as meaning as if all the façade has been stripped away.'

'All the trappings of "being a counsellor", if that is what you mean.'

'Hmm, yes.'

'I am a counsellor still, but I am actually more of a person. And that is why I like to think of myself as person-centred rather than client-centred, even though I know that client-centred is the phrase used to describe the person-centred approach applied to counselling and psychotherapy.'

'Hmm, so you prefer to see yourself as person-centred.'

'Yes, the person of the client and the person of myself. Two persons. In those really human moments that's all we have and all we are. And yes, I bring my professional counsellorism into it – I know that's not a word – but I am there fundamentally as a person because it is me as a person in my affect, in the way I am touched by my client, and the way that I respond, that contributes to the healing process.'

'Your presence as a person?'

'Yes, my presence as a person, and I would focus it even more and say that it is something about the heart of me, as a person, that is the focus for the healing.'

Quality of presence is a concept that infers that there is something about the presence of the therapist, when they are functioning fully and effectively within the therapeutic relationship, that creates an opportunity for movement to occur within the client. Rogers wrote 'when I am at my best, as a group facilitator or as a therapist, I discover another characteristic. I find that when I am closest to the intuitive self, when I am somewhat in touch with the unknown in me, when perhaps I am in a slightly altered state of consciousness, then whatever I do seems to be full of healing. Then, simply my *presence* is releasing and helpful to the other' (Rogers, 1980, p. 29).

He describes this process in terms of being a 'transcendent phenomena' and makes reference to 'inner spirit'. Whether we want to use terms such as this or not, he pointed at some level or way of being that seemed to have a particularly significant effect. It was Emerson in his essay 'Social Aims', who wrote, 'Don't *say* things. What you *are* stands over you the while, and thunders so that I cannot hear what you say to the contrary' (Emerson, 1987, p. 450). Elsewhere, from one of a series of spiritual teachings we read that, 'one may disguise the tone of voice, but the radiation of the heart cannot be falsified' (Agni Yoga Society, 1959, p. 31). As the therapist tends towards a more complete presence and engagement with the client, perhaps a shift occurs in the relationship, in consciousness, in some manner that the psychological theoreticians cannot quantify but which the mystics have known down the ages. And that shift has something to do with the opening of the heart to another.

'Your presence, but more particularly the presence of, and the response, of your heart is what contributes to some kind of healing process?'
'I think so.'
'Interesting. Something about there being a heartfelt response, or am I projecting my meaning into your understanding?'
'It has to be heartfelt. Otherwise it is false. And there is something about my clients – and I am sure not only them – but it takes me to a place where all I have to offer is myself, and the key part of myself that I have to offer is my heart.'

What does 'heartfelt responding' mean in the context of the therapeutic relationship and person-centred theory? Is the heart another sense, another system through which we can apprehend the world around us? We certainly feel experiences in the heart, it seems to be a receptive organ in some mysterious way. And can it give out as well, as though the therapist needs to be able to function through the heart in their relationship with their client for the psychotherapeutic endeavour to have real meaning? And when we work with clients, such as Ania, who touch our hearts deeply, what occurs in those moments of heartfelt responding, and what effect does it have on the client and the counsellor? And what processes in supervision ensure that the heart of the therapist is prepared for their next encounter in therapeutic relationship?

It is perhaps another language in which to explore the application of the person-centred approach, and perhaps a language particularly pertinent to clients who, through their experiences in life, may be evidencing a state or way of being that might encompass something of the phenomenon of feeling, or being, heart-broken.

Points for discussion

- What has the supervision session left you thinking and feeling?
- Do you believe Debbie has raised all the issues that needed to be raised?
- How effective do you think Rob is as a supervisor from what you have read? Is his supervisory approach consistent with person-centred practice?
- Do you think that there is a 'raw will to live' within each of us that circumstances force into emergence?
- What are your thoughts about the notion of 'pseudocongruence' alluded to in the supervision session?
- Should person-centred counsellors accept information about a client from an assessment made by someone else? What are the pros and cons of this in your experience?
- Is 'authentic living' an acceptable goal of therapy? Does this fit comfortably with person-centred principles?
- Critically evaluate Debbie's responses to Ania on the phone. Were they appropriate and consistent with person-centred practice?
- Write supervision notes for this session from the standpoint of Rob, and that of Debbie.

CHAPTER 4

Counselling session 4: the counsellor's congruence is challenged

Ania was in the waiting area. She had arrived before the appointment time. She noticed a poster on the wall, it was for an afternoon for people from Bosnia, an opportunity to meet people, make new friends, or just spend an afternoon. Children welcome. It appealed. She hadn't made many friends in England. The agency that had brought her over had put her in touch with people from her country, and she met up with some of them, but she was more interested in spending time with Maria. But there was something about the poster's wording that appealed. She noted down the time and the phone number for information.

She heard her name. It was Debbie's voice. 'Hi Ania, ready to come through?'

'Yes, hello Debbie, I was reading this poster. I could go to that.'

'Yes, I understand it has just started. It takes place here once a week. Very friendly. They play music and, well, it's an opportunity to connect and for people to perhaps speak their own language. I think it is very good.'

'I would like that, and Maria would meet new people as well. It says children are welcome.'

'Yes, it is very much a family afternoon.'

'Do I need to ask someone to come?'

'You can let Julie know at the desk, she will pass your interest on, and then just turn up.'

'I will think about it. Thank you.'

They went into the counselling room.

'So, how are things, Ania, how is Maria? I am very aware that when you called on the phone last week things were not easy.'

> Is this directive? It has given the start of the session a focus, but it is also conveying unconditional positive regard towards Ania and her daughter, which is also important. It is reasonable that a client might expect such an enquiry. It raises an interesting question. Omitting to ask something at the start of a session might communicate a lack of empathy, warmth or

unconditional positive regard to a client who reasonably expects an enquiry as a result of something that has happened since the last meeting.

However, it would be inappropriate to ask about Maria if the phone call and cancellation of the previous session had not occurred.

'No, it was not good. But Maria is much better now. Thank you. She has drawn another picture for you. Ania took the picture from out of her bag. It is of you and me. I told her what you look like. I hope you like it.'

Debbie looked at the picture that Ania gave her. It had two people sitting in a room, with a table and the window and the orange curtains. And the green chairs.

'You have described the room to her.'

'Yes, and she would like to see it. Perhaps if we come to the afternoon, if the room is not in use, perhaps she could see? And she wants to see you as well.'

'That would be fine. If the door is open then I am free, if it is closed I have a client with me.'

'I will explain to Maria. Thank you.'

Debbie felt very touched by what Ania was saying. Maria was clearly alive to what was going on around her and for her mother. She wondered just how much she must pick up from her mother's sadness as well, however much Ania tried to keep it from her. She knew how sensitive children were, she knew how sensitive her own were. When she'd gone through a difficult period a few years back they just sort of were there for her, not really saying anything, but they just always seemed to appear and be around when she was upset. They had talked about it since and they had said that they knew that she was sad and that they wanted to try to make her happy again. She knew she felt quite emotional as thoughts arose briefly in her mind. But it did not feel appropriate to say anything about it.

'So, how do you want to use our time this afternoon, Ania?'

'I'm not sure. It was not easy after the last session and I wondered if this was helping me. But I know I have to do this. I just feel so sensitive, particularly loud noises and places where there are lots of people. I just feel very anxious at the moment.'

'More so than previously?'

'I think so.'

'So loud, sudden noises and places with lots of people, you feel very anxious.'

'I want to get away, to leave those places.'

'To get away.'

'To go home. I either want to go home, or go to the park, when it is quiet. I like to sit and watch Maria play, and feed the pigeons. But if there are too many people around then I want to go home.'

'It seems that you are very sensitive to too much happening around you.'

'Or something loud and unexpected. Like the noise here that time.'

Debbie nodded, 'yes.'

'I do not feel safe when there is noise and too many people.'

'Mhmm, and it has got worse.'

'Yes. I think so. But I have to go out. But I have to feel safe.'

'And if you do not feel safe then you have to leave, get away, go somewhere else.'

'That is right.'

'That can't be easy.'

'No, it is not.'

Debbie was struck by how the dialogue had become rather question and answer, it felt quite stilted. She wasn't sure whether this might be a language issue, or simply how Ania was feeling at the moment, not wanting to say very much for fear, perhaps, of where it might lead. It felt like she was perhaps speaking this way in order to keep control.

'And I guess it makes it difficult to feel in control when it is like that.'

> This proves to be a therapeutically helpful response drawn from feelings that have arisen in the counsellor through the relational process with the client. It is therefore an appropriate expression of congruence.

'I like to be in control. Too many bad things have happened, too many things that I have had no control over.'

Debbie felt the atmosphere change, she sensed that Ania was holding an awareness of some of those bad things now, in this moment.

'Too many things, bad things, where you did not have any control.'

Ania shook her head and looked down. 'You have no control of bombs, where they will land, where you should be.'

'No, no, not knowing where they will land.'

> The counsellor has not empathised with 'control' in this response, although the earlier comment may suffice as the client will know that the counsellor has an appreciation of the 'control' issue.

'It is a terrible thing to be under attack like that, in your own home, not knowing, but fearing. Trying to live your life, but not knowing.'

'Not knowing . . .' Debbie picked up on the not knowing which Ania had repeated.

'You want to believe everything will be OK, that you will be OK, that those you love will be OK, but it is not necessarily so.'

'No, no. You want to believe, you try to believe, but bad things happen.'

'I do not believe people understand, unless they have sat there, hearing the explosions, waiting, just waiting.'

> Is the client actually saying, 'your responses tell me that you do not understand'? It is an important moment. The counsellor must be genuine in her response if she is to respond to that sensed question, though it is not a

question that has been directly verbalised. The counsellor must make a decision. The risk is that she may end up sounding defensive or justifying something about herself.

'I would not pretend to understand, Ania, but I can hear what you tell me about it, I can appreciate something of the feelings. I was not there but I can feel it now as you tell me. But I know I cannot fully understand what it is like.'

The counsellor puts the focus on herself and not on what the client is communicating. There is no empathy to the concern expressed by the client. It is valid what Debbie has said, but is it therapeutically helpful? She could have said, 'people have to have been there, sat there, hearing the explosions, and waiting, endless waiting' which would have empathised and ended with strong focus on what Ania's statement had lead up to – that sense of forever waiting.

It is not that Debbie's response was wrong, it's what would have felt appropriate for her to say in the experience of the therapeutic relationship. It can be of value, though, to consider the possibility of other responses that could have more therapeutic value, or perhaps a different therapeutic value.

'I would not want you to. For you to understand you would have had to have experienced it, and I would not want that.'
'Thank you, Ania.' Debbie lapsed into silence, unsure what to say next.
'For me, it was what you had to get used to.'
'Yes. Something that you had to get used to, there was no choice.'
'There was no choice. You did what you had to do. Life had to go on.' She stopped abruptly. Thinking of her parents whose life had not gone on, whose life had been destroyed in one explosive moment. She was not feeling so sad about it at that moment, her jaw was set. She was angry. She was angry that they were dead, killed by those bastard Serbs. She was angry that her parents were not alive to share in Maria's life. She was angry that those responsible had not been punished.
'You look angry, Ania, a lot to feel angry about.'
'I get very angry, Debbie, and then I get sad. I think about Maria, not having a grandpapa or a grandmama, and it makes me angry and sad.'
Debbie noted that it was Maria's loss, and her reaction to Maria's loss that she was describing, not her own direct loss associated with the death of her parents.
'It makes you angry and sad thinking about what Maria will not have.'

In spite of what Debbie noted, she has maintained empathy for what Ania has said. This is important. She has not directed Ania's focus away from what she is experiencing.

Yes, people do divert feelings of loss from themselves on to others. It is a way of coping, of keeping some of their own feelings contained. It is not something that the person-centred counsellor would challenge. It is how it is, how the client needs to be, and it is accepted.

This is an area where person-centred counselling may be seen to differ from other theoretical approaches that would perhaps more readily encourage the challenging of this displacement of feelings. From a person-centred perspective the client has established a way of being that works for her. To disturb it when the client is not expressing any reason or motivation to do so would be to threaten part of her psychological support system. The client is not ready for this. From a person-centred perspective it would be abusive to challenge and disturb Ania's way of being.

'She is a little girl, she should have that. It is not right that she does not.'
'Not right that Maria does not have a grandpapa or a grandmama.'
'She only has me.'
'She only has you, her mother.'
'And I only have her.'
'Yes, you only have her, it feels like you only have each other.'
'I think she will make new friends as she grows up. She will not have to know what I know. She will be free to live her own life. I hope so. That is how I want it to be.'
'Yes, that is important to you, that she does grow up and make new friends and be free to live her own life.'
'Very important. She must not have to think of the things that I have to think about.'
'You would not want her to have the thoughts that you have.'
'Or the feelings.'
'No, or the feelings.'
Ania lapsed into silence herself. She had to protect Maria. She did not have to know about the terrible things that had happened. She must be sure not to let her know. It was not right that she should have to know. But she must know to hate the Serbs. It was not easy to make sense of. She wanted Maria not to know of the terrible things, but she had to know some things, but not yet, not now, maybe later when she was older.
'Why do you do this? Why do you give your time to listen to people like me?'
The question seemed to come out of the blue, and Debbie was momentarily taken aback. It felt like it intruded in her own attempt to be with Ania, with what was on her mind as she spoke about protecting Maria.
'I want to help. I think that counselling does help. I want to offer a space and a relationship where you feel accepted and able to say what you want or be how you need to be. I want to try and help people to cope, to maybe make sense of the things that have happened to them but only if that is what the person wants. It is up to the person I am with.'

'There is no sense to the things that happened. There can be no sense. We were
    victims of actions that should not have happened. There is no sense to be made
    of it.'
'Perhaps that is partly what makes it so difficult.'

The counsellor has responded to a direct question, and the client has then
picked up on part of her response. The client is responding to something
that the counsellor has introduced, but it is because it has resonated with
something held deeply by the client. It is, perhaps, unwittingly directive
although the client was free to pick up on anything said by the therapist.
However, the final response above is not empathic. It is the counsellor now
trying to make sense of what is being experienced by the client. It could be
argued, therefore, that the counsellor has a driving need to make sense of
things and this is a supervision issue. It is not a response reflecting person-
centred working. However, whether it will actually disturb or derail the flow
of experiencing and expression within the client remains to be seen.

'For me, no. It is what those people do. I do not need to make sense of it, they are
    stupid and evil. I have to live my life, I have no need to make sense of them.'
Debbie was struck again by the forcefulness and the hatred towards those who
    had perpetrated the violence upon Ania and her family, and in truth she was
    not surprised although there seemed something incongruent about hearing
    Ania speak that way. Yet it was Ania and she must accept that this
    was as much part of Ania as was the devoted mother and the saddened daugh-
    ter, and no doubt the traumatised sister as well. She must accept all aspects,
    all parts, of Ania. She could not, and should not, give any impression of
    favouring any part. They all existed – and there would be others, no doubt –
    all deserving of being heard, understood, and to experience the presence of the
    therapeutic conditions. Whilst she might conceive of them in certain terms,
    what was more important was how Ania would experience them, which
    might be quite different.

Whilst a person-centred counsellor might see a client in this way, they
would not introduce it, and certainly not give them names. It may be
an aid to appreciating the complexities and dynamics of the client, but
that is all it can be. And it may not reflect the way the client experiences
themselves.

   With regard to the counsellor's sense of the client's incongruence, this is
surely arising out of the counsellor's own incongruence. She is projecting
expectation as to how the client will be. There is perhaps a resistance, in
that moment, to accepting the client as an angry and unforgiving woman.

'You do not need to make sense of the stupid and evil people. You have to live your life.'

'I hope they burn in hell.' The words were spoken with a venomous fire.

'You want to see them burn in hell.'

'I would like to see *them*, I would like to see the terror in *their* eyes. I would like to see *them* suffer. It is what they deserve.'

'They deserve to burn and you would like to see it, see their terror, their suffering.'

Ania felt strong as she had these thoughts. They were good thoughts to have. She believed in heaven and hell, her Christian faith was important to her. She believed God would punish them, but she wanted them to suffer on earth as well. She did not want to forgive them, they were beyond being forgiven. God would understand that. She knew God would understand that. People like that made Him angry.

'Can you understand how I feel? I don't think you can.'

'I don't think I can, but I do experience the anger in you as you speak, the desire for retribution and punishment.'

'But you do not think it is how it should be. You want me to forgive them.'

Ouch, thought Debbie, yes I do because without forgiveness the cycle of violence continues, but what to say. She couldn't hesitate, and she knew she was already hesitating.

This is a critical moment in the session and in the therapeutic relationship.

'I don't think it is easy to forgive people when they cause such pain and suffering. And it is not for me to say what people should, or should not do.' Damn thought Debbie, too many words. Be simple, be straight. Say it as it is. 'I would like to see forgiveness, but not now, not yet.'

'Thank you for your honesty. That is important to me. I do not agree with you, but I appreciate you being honest. I think you would feel different if you were me.'

'I think I probably would as well, but I do not know, and I am not you, I can only feel what I feel as me.'

'Do you accept how I feel?'

'Yes, yes I do.'

'I believe you, I see it on your face. If I did not see it there I would leave.'

The degree to which the previous critical moment was significant is revealed. Ania is picking up on Debbie's way of being, she is challenging her, checking her out. It was crucially important that Debbie was honest in her response. Her eyes would therefore reflect the truth of what she was saying. It is absolutely vital that counsellors are congruent. Yes, it may not be possible all of the time, but it should be at least most of the time – and increasingly so – and certainly in moments such as these.

'I am struck by the strength in your voice, Ania, these are very important things for you, and for me. If I could not accept what you feel, I would want to resolve that, and if I could not then you should find someone else who did accept your feelings.'

' "Resolve?", please explain.'

'Mhmm, to sort out, make clear, find a way so that I could accept your feelings.'

'I understand.'

Debbie was still very much struck by the strength in Ania's voice. Why was she so surprised? Here was a woman who had faced traumatic loss and atrocity perpetrated on herself and her brother, and no doubt friends and her people in general, who had survived, given birth to her daughter and had come to another country, and devoted herself to caring for her and bringing her up. This was Ania the survivor speaking, Ania, proud Croatian mother who was going to survive.

'You are a strong woman, Ania, a proud Croatian mother.'

'I do not feel strong sometimes,' Ania looked down, but looked up again as she added, 'but I am proud'.

Debbie nodded as she saw the look in Ania's eyes, and the strength that whilst Ania might not be owning in this moment, she, Debbie, could see as being present. 'I am pleased to know you, Ania. I feel I have learned much about you today.'

'And I about you, Debbie.'

The session drew slowly to a close, the remainder of the session Ania talked about the family group at the centre, and asked more about what it was like. Debbie answered as best she could, and they agreed that Ania should leave the session a little early to talk to Julie about it. Then she wouldn't be delayed and risk missing the bus home as she had to be back on time for the childminder.

Points for discussion

- Can you accept Ania's feelings – really accept them? If not, what would you do if Ania was your client?
- Critically evaluate Debbie's application of the person-centred approach in this session. Were there key person-centred responses and, if so, which and to what effect?
- How did you interpret Ania's 'stilted' responses as you were reading them? Were they a language difficulty, self-protection or something else?
- How might you have responded to Ania's statement, 'but you do not think it is how it should be. You want me to forgive them.'?
- If you were Debbie, what might you be taking to supervision from this session other than that indicated in the text. Explain your answer and what would you hope to achieve?
- Write counselling notes for this session.

CHAPTER 5

Counselling session 5: Ania tells her story

'I wish to tell you more about the events that led up to me coming to England. I want you to know, I want you to understand.' Ania was sitting quite stiffly in her chair, but with a very purposeful and matter of fact air about her. 'I have been thinking about last week, and I feel it is important that you know and you understand, as best you can, what happened in Bosnia which I call my country because I lived there, though as you know I am Croatian.'

'Yes, I do appreciate that and I want to say that I do wish to understand.'

> Clients often will want to tell their story – sometimes it will be in the first session, sometimes they will need to feel safe in themselves and with the counsellor and it will take longer before they begin to talk in this way. It is an important step, a critical time. The person-centred counsellor needs to be at their best. The client is giving of themselves. They need to speak and they need someone to bear witness to what they have to say. The core conditions must be offered. Sometimes the counsellor will say very little, the client will keep talking. Their need to talk is more important in that moment than their need to check that they have been heard. Perhaps they accept that because the counsellor is there, in the room, offering attention. For other clients they will need to know that the counsellor has heard them. The story may last a whole session or more, or a short period of time, but when the time is right the client is likely to be feeling a need to tell it. This must be respected.

'The war was terrible. Villages and families torn apart. Neighbours fighting neighbours, marriages split, it was as if the whole country was at war with itself, and, of course, there was Serbia who caused it all in the first place.'

Debbie did not know all the details of the causes of the war, and was not going to get into a discussion over the facts. Her role was to accept the perspective that her client had, to listen to what was real for her.

'It seemed chaotic from what we learned here.'

'It was chaotic, very chaotic. And the Muslims, of course, were killed and treated very badly as well. Many thousands were rounded up. It was terrible. I am not a Muslim but I had Muslim friends, and I do not know what became of them, even if they are still alive,' she paused and swallowed, her eyes welling with tears, 'but I do not believe any people should be treated like that, just because they are different.'

Debbie nodded, she agreed, but it was not her role to agree, but to empathise. 'You were friends with Muslim people and you do not believe that the Muslims should have been treated so badly.' Debbie paused briefly, then picked up on the tears in Ania's eyes. 'It saddens you greatly what happened.'

Ania nodded and continued with her story. 'After my parents were killed my brother, Tomas, came home. He was in the police force and lived in another region. It was agreed that I would go and live with him, at least for a while. There was nothing left of our home, not really, just a few possessions remained, which we took. We were going to make a new start. I had relatives in Croatia but we wanted to stay in Bosnia. It was where we had lived all our lives and where we wanted to stay.'

'So you went with your brother, nothing really left to stay for in the town.'

'That is right. The fighting continued, and it was bad. People were being rounded up and shot. Women taken away, particularly Muslim women and raped. It seemed like the world had forgotten us, that no one wanted to know, no one wanted to help. It was a terrible time, we all feared for our lives, everyone. We had good friends in Bosnia, but we were Croatian and we knew that we might have to return to Croatia. In fact, we were beginning to make plans to return and to stay with an aunt and uncle for a while close to Zagreb.'

'You really feared for your lives.'

'Yes, and we were right to, Debbie. It was not safe, we were not safe, but we did not know how unsafe we were. If we had known, we would have left before, and Tomas would be alive.' Ania's voice started to go weak as she spoke the last sentence.

'Take your time, Ania, there is no hurry, take your time.' She did not empathise with what had been said, she felt there was no need. Ania wanted to tell her story. Her role would be to, in effect, listen and bear witness to the tragic events that she wanted, needed to describe. Debbie waited for Ania to continue.

Ania swallowed. Her feelings were very present. She had looked down as she sought to compose herself a little before continuing. But she couldn't, she could feel herself becoming weak as the images returned, the sounds, the awful sounds, what they did to her, what they did to him. It wasn't that it was only now coming to the surface, the memories were with her daily, but she fought them and put her energy into Maria. The love she had for her daughter was what mattered to her. Conceived in violence she was determined to love her. Maria would live and she would know, one day, what had happened. She would be strong. She would stand as a proud Croatian and perhaps return back to her country – one day.

The images fought to assert themselves within her tortured mind. She swallowed. 'They came in the night. There were just the two of us in the house. We heard the vehicles and the sudden crash of the door being broken down. We were upstairs. Tomas made me run, said he'd try and delay them so I could get away. He had a gun that he kept with him at all times. I heard the shouting as I tried to run away from the house. I heard the gun being fired. They saw me and dragged me back.' She could hear the voices in her head, the shouts. Yet she felt somehow distant in herself. 'They raped me, forced me down in the dust outside. Tomas was held and made to watch. They were beating him as well. I remember hearing him shout to me, "I love you."' It felt to her as though she was strangely distant as she re-lived the events. 'They took me to where I could see him, they were still beating him, kicking him, hitting him with their guns. One of them took ...' The distance left her, she was there, it was real, it felt like it was happening again. She saw the knife, more like a machete, it glistened momentarily in the headlights from the vehicle nearby. She broke down in tears, deep, heart-wrenching sobs that burned through her body. She was shaking, Debbie got up and went over to her, holding her as she continued to cry. 'If I had that knife I would kill them, kill them all, very slowly.' The pain had turned to anger. 'They held him down and forced me to watch, holding my head so I could see. They cut off his right hand, saying something that it was the last time he would fire a gun at a Serb.' The tears were hot in her eyes on her face, but she was determined to keep talking. 'He was brave, Oh God he was brave.' She swallowed, the lump hot and hard in her throat. 'He told them he'd shoot with his other hand. They cut that off as well and left him lying there, laughing as he bled and writhed in pain. Then they raped me again. He was screaming in pain and then I heard a single shot, and there was silence.' She was clinging to Debbie. 'I don't know for how long, I must have lost consciousness. They must have left, I don't know. I don't remember much more. I have vague memories, waking up, and I don't know, I don't know. I-I don't know ...'

Debbie held Ania against her. She didn't know what to say. What was there to say? Her heart was going out to her, it ached. There were no words. 'No, you don't know ...'

Ania said nothing, she felt utterly drained of energy and numb, a strange kind of numbness, and a creeping coldness at the core of her being. She could feel Debbie holding her and it felt good – someone to hold on to. Ania clung to her amidst waves of emotion – hate, despair, sadness, horror. She wasn't thinking these words. But they were components of the raw pain that she felt, not just in her head, her heart, it was in her whole body. She burned and yet felt numb. But she knew she must keep talking. She had to finish the story. It was important in spite of all that she was feeling. She let go her grip.

'I was at the hospital. They were very good. They looked after me. They told me that when I was brought in I was carrying Tomas's right hand. I don't remember that. I must have carried it with me. I am glad I did that, Debbie. I hope that hand killed some of them before they reached him. They have never found his body. His hand is buried in a church.' Ania felt her distancing from the feelings and the events returning. She relaxed her hold on Debbie, who reciprocated.

Ania took tissues from the box and wiped her eyes, dried her face and blew her nose. 'That is what happened, Debbie, that is what those animals did.'

Debbie nodded. 'I feel horrified, humbled, cold, numb having heard what you have said, and I don't have the words ... But you have experienced atrocity that no human-being should be subject to. But you were, and I salute your courage in telling me and I am glad you have told me, Ania.' Debbie spoke from her heart. This slightly built woman in front of her had survived an ordeal that no one should have to face. 'You have every right to think and feel everything that you do, Ania.' Debbie wanted to affirm her acceptance of all that Ania felt, and of her right to feel it.

'I wanted you to know, Debbie. I am sorry if it was painful.'

'It was painful, but my pain is as nothing to yours, or Tomas'.' She felt she wanted to mention him, to have not done so would not feel right. Whatever mental and emotional state was Ania in when she had come round? No body, maybe just a hand left in the dust. She knew she had no concept of what that was like, totally beyond her own horizon of experience.

'I will never forgive them, Debbie, and I will never forget. And Maria must know, will know, one day ... one day.'

Debbie felt her jaw tighten. She could appreciate why Ania did not want the memory to be lost, but she knew how it would pass the horror on to another generation and perhaps perpetuate the ancient hatreds that might flare up at a future time. But that was her reaction, and not for her to comment on.

'You don't want the memory to be lost, it is not something you want to forgive or forget ...'

'I will never forget, never.' Ania spoke strongly and fiercely, cutting across Debbie before she could finish speaking.

'Never, never forget.'

'And I must live my life. I have Maria.'

'Mhmm, yes, you have a life and you have Maria.'

'She is named after my ..., after our mother.'

Debbie smiled slightly and nodded.

Ania looked at Debbie as a sudden rush of emotion washed through her, a sudden moment of extreme vulnerability and uncertainty, perhaps as a result of the emotional release that had just taken place. 'Oh Debbie, how will it be for us?' The tears were welling up in her eyes again.

'For you and for Maria, in the future?'

Debbie nodded, and sniffed, reaching over for another tissue. 'I don't want to stay here, I want to go back, back home, when it is safe. I do not know that it is safe, but I want to. It is my country. I still have relatives but I have not been back. I want to but I am scared to.' She went silent and looked down.

Debbie had returned to her seat. 'Want to but scared to, Ania, so want to go back, but ...'

'One day, but when and how will it be? Sometimes I try not to think too much for the future. It is enough to think about today, and tomorrow, but there are times when I try to look ahead ...' She looked up. 'I cannot. I do not know.'

'You do not know what lies ahead, how it will be, where you will be.'

'Perhaps I will meet a nice Englishman who will take care of me.' She smiled and looked slightly embarrassed.

'Perhaps you might, Ania, perhaps you might.'

'But I am sure I would still want to go home and, well, he might not want that.'

'Mhmm, makes it hard to imagine the future if you still wanted to go home.'

'I suppose I will have to decide where I want to be, and I know I want to go home, one day.'

'One day . . .'

'I have decided we will go to the afternoon and meet the other people from Bosnia. It will be good for Maria. I want her to meet more of her own people. We will be able to talk in our own language, that will be good for Maria as well. She knows a little. She needs to improve her language for the future.'

'It seems like you are really thinking this through and planning ahead, and whilst I realise you are saying it is uncertain, it feels like you are preparing to return to Bosnia, or Croatia, at some point.'

'You are right. I think I am.'

The session continued with Ania saying a little more about Maria. She also talked a bit more about Bosnia and her people, what it had been like before the war. Ania left the session looking forward to meeting people from Bosnia. She knew how it was with people from her country. There was a lot of friendliness. It was the war that had torn things apart. She had to move on. She had to. She had Maria to think about. She was also glad to have told Debbie. In a way, she knew she didn't want her to have to hear it, but she also knew she had to tell it, really tell it. She hadn't said so much when the other lady had assessed her. She didn't feel she wanted to, it was all questions and she had not felt comfortable. But it had become important to her for Debbie to know, to understand.

Debbie sat quietly after the session. She did feel numb still, slightly spaced out as she thought about what Ania had told her. Ania, the woman sitting opposite her and who had faced those awful actions perpetrated on her and her brother. A woman who, by outward appearances, could be any woman, but Ania carried a set of experiences that in some way set her apart. At least, that was what Debbie felt, and then she questioned her attitude. Who was she to categorise? Surely it was up to Ania to decide whether she felt apart? So many women were raped, so many people tortured and killed in that region, perhaps it was she, Debbie, who was set apart, apart from those experiences herself?

And she loves Maria, a child conceived in the midst of horror and death. Debbie struggled with that. She wondered if Ania's intense love for Maria masked something else, something hidden and deeper. But she knew that was fruitless speculation. The reality that she experienced from Ania was that of love and devotion and that was what she would accept until or unless something changed or something different emerged. No point in looking for ghosts that are not necessarily there, she thought to herself. But she was left wondering, nevertheless. She shook her head, no, Ania is surviving as only she knows how, and Maria is a crucial part of that. They are somehow facing something together, though only Ania knows really what it is.

She sat back in the chair. She needed a cool drink and some fresh air, and time to clear herself. Clear herself . . . What did that mean? Try to get herself back into a place where she could accurately empathise with her next client, where memories from the previous session did not intrude, where her congruent experiences and responses were pertinent to the session. She took up her pen and began to write notes for the session. On another piece of paper she wrote out the feelings and thoughts that were present for her, feeling a need to express them in some way, get them out of her system. She looked at the list. Yes, and the depth of my feelings are as nothing compared to those of Ania was the thought that struck her.

Points for discussion

- If you were listing your thoughts and feelings in response to Ania, what would you write?
- What might make it difficult for you to listen to Ania speak about the traumatic events she described?
- Consider Debbie's responses. Would yours have been similar? How might you have reacted differently, and why?
- What aspects of the person-centred approach do you believe are particularly significant when working therapeutically with clients who have experienced atrocities of this kind?
- How do you react to Debbie's speculations after the session?
- Write notes for this session.

CHAPTER 6

Counselling session 6: Maria attends with Ania

Ania was due and Debbie went out to the waiting room, but she had not yet arrived. She returned to the counselling room to wait. It was not like Ania to be late. When she had not arrived at a previous session she had called. Debbie hoped she was OK. She could hear voices and it sounded like Ania apologising for being late. Debbie got up and went out to see. Yes it was Ania, and she was not alone.

Ania turned as Debbie approached.

'Hello. Sorry I'm late. I have brought Maria. I hope that is OK. The childminder cancelled late and, well, this seemed the best thing to do. And Maria has been wanting to meet you.'

'That's OK.' Debbie squatted down. 'Hello, Maria. I'm Debbie. It's so nice to meet you.'

Maria hesitated, caught between stepping back behind her mama's skirt, and coming forward to the woman that her mama came to see each week.

'You're not usually shy.'

'Never mind.' Debbie paused. 'Hello, Maria.'

'She's brought a picture for you.'

'I'd like to see that. Come on, let's go through and Maria, you can see the room that mama comes to each week.'

Maria's curiosity won and she walked forward.

Debbie got up and led the way. She wasn't surprised that Maria had come. She had accepted long ago that these situations arose, and she accepted that sometimes it was for the best for the child to come as well.

Debbie was aware that there wasn't another chair for Maria, but there was a large cushion in the corner which she moved over for Maria to sit on if she wanted to. Maria, however, chose to clamber on to her mother's lap, and sat with her head against Ania's chest, looking across at Debbie, but clearly holding her mother.

'Not like you to be shy, Masza.' Ania always called Maria this, though when talking to other people she called her Maria.

Maria said nothing.

'It's a new environment.' Debbie spoke to Ania, then turned her attention to Maria. 'It's really nice to have you here, Maria, and mama says you have a picture for me, but I will leave it for you to decide if you want to show it to me. I would love to see it when you are ready.' She smiled.

Maria looked back, and then looked at her mother.

'I have it in my bag, Masza.'

Maria stayed in Ania's lap. 'I'm sure she will show it to you later.'

Debbie nodded as she looked towards Maria, and then looked back to Ania, and smiled warmly. 'So, obviously it will perhaps seem a little different with Maria here with us.'

'Yes, it could not be helped. It was this or cancel, but I did want to come and tell you about the meeting I went to and, well, Maria asked if she could come. I told her that I did not know, but it was all at the last minute and so I brought her with me. She's quiet now but she has been wanting to meet you.'

'Well, I am pleased to meet Maria.' Debbie again looked at Maria and smiled.

'I am very proud of her, Debbie, she is my little Masza.' Ania kissed her on the head and gave her a hug.

Debbie smiled and eased back a little in the chair. She realised she had been sitting forward and had a bit of tension in her shoulders.

'So, what do you want to talk about, Ania?'

'The group. We really enjoyed ourselves, didn't we, Masza?'

Maria nodded.

'Mhmm, so it was really good to go to.'

'It was. It was good to speak in my own language and to talk to people who knew places and, well, just knew how it had been.'

Debbie nodded, having a sense of how important that can be for people, but clearly how important it was for Ania. 'Sense of shared knowledge.'

'Yes, knowledge and, yes, and it was very friendly. And there were other children as well, which was good. So we shall go again next week and we will continue to go there, won't we?' She gave Maria a squeeze, who nodded and smiled.

Debbie smiled and waited to see what Ania would want to say next.

Maria leaned up and whispered to Ania. Debbie did not hear what she said.

'Yes, of course you can.' She looked to Debbie. 'She wants to show you her picture now.'

'I would love to see it, Maria.'

Maria scrambled off her mother's lap as Ania leant over to take it from her bag. Maria took it and brought it over to Debbie who now leaned forward to take it.

'Thank you Maria. Can you tell me about it?' She turned it towards herself, there was a picture of a tall woman and a little girl – she guessed it was of Maria and Ania, and they were holding hands, and both smiling.

'Mama and me. It is in the kitchen. I like it in the kitchen.'

'Mhmm, you like being in the kitchen with your mama.'

'Yes. And that ...' Maria was standing next to Debbie and was pointing to the picture, 'that's the table where we sit and eat, and that's the window.'

'It's a very nice picture, Maria, you and mama in the kitchen, and the table and the window.'

Maria smiled, and looked back at Ania.

'She drew it for you, Debbie. She said she wanted to draw a picture of us for you.'

'For me, to have?'

Maria nodded.

'Thank you. I am very happy, Maria, thank you.' Debbie paused. 'I would like to take it home and put it on my kitchen wall. Would you like that?'

Maria thought about it. 'Yes, then you can think about mama and me when you eat.'

'I would like that, Maria, thank you.' She paused. 'Let me put it here on the table for now where it will be safe.'

Maria looked very pleased, and she went over to her mother.

'Do you want your colouring book? You can sit on the cushion; mama and Debbie need to talk for a while.'

Maria nodded. She was pleased that Debbie had liked her picture and was going to put it in her kitchen and think of them. She took the book and some crayons, and settled herself down.

'Hope you don't mind her being here.'

'It is lovely to meet her, Ania. I know it will make the session different today, but that is OK.'

'I would not normally bring her but, well, it seemed for the best.'

'Yes, yes. It is OK. You did what you felt best, and it became an opportunity for me and Maria to meet each other, and for her to see where you come.'

Childcare arrangements can be problematic and the situation that has arisen can occur. How does a person-centred counsellor respond? As a one-off it seems acceptable for Maria to come into the session. Yes, it will change the dynamic and the content, but it may have other therapeutic benefits.

If it started to become a regular occurrence then a discussion would be necessary as to how to best proceed, with possible re-negotiation of the counselling arrangements and liaison with the social worker and maybe the health visitors, to see what other arrangements could be made.

'I showed her the room – well, the door was closed so she saw the door, when we came to the group here.'

'And it seems like it was really good.'

'Yes.' Ania lapsed into silence, she was looking over to Maria, who was concentrating on her colouring, seemingly quite oblivious to the conversation her mama was having with Debbie.

'She really does like drawing and colouring. She's wonderful.'

'Yes.' Debbie smiled.

'It is difficult for me to know what to talk about. I don't want to get upset this week with Maria here.'

'No, I understand. Is there anything you want to talk about, Ania?'

'I suppose I want to understand a little more about how counselling will help me. I know it is helping me. I am pleased to be here, and to know you, Debbie. I will never forget the past, but I want to be able to face the future.'
Debbie nodded. 'It is about facing the future, yes?'
'I met with people and, well, no one really talked about the things that happened to them. They talked about good times and their hopes. I did not know what to say. I do not know what my future will be. That made me sad. But it will not stop me going. It is important for Maria, and for me.'
Debbie nodded again. 'Hearing their hopes made you aware of not knowing what your future would be like.'
'No. I am sure I will talk about the past another time. But I do not know my future. I have Maria, she is my future for now, for many years. But she will go to school and I must work. Or perhaps I should return to my country. I want Maria to speak our language and I am concerned she will not learn it so well here.'
'So you see your future back in Bosnia …'
'No, I think we will go to Croatia, to Zagreb, and perhaps it is something I should begin to plan for soon.'
'You feel you should start planning to return?'
'It is difficult for me. I think so, but I do not know.'
'Mhmm, yes, you think you want to plan to return but you cannot be sure, yes?'
'How can I be sure?'
Debbie nodded, the words triggered her memory of a song, the following line "in a world that's constantly changing …" 'Yes, so many things to consider?'

These things happen. The counsellor notes it, sets it aside and maintains focus on the client. There is a truth and a relevance to what the counsellor has remembered, and it has disturbed the empathic flow as she has responded to the focus on the 'many things to consider' rather than the 'how can I be sure?'.

'Yes, but then, well, I suppose I do not know what is for the best, but I think I must return. It will be difficult for Maria, she must make a big adjustment, but the longer I leave it the more difficult it will be for her.'
'So, it is your concern for Maria that is important, that it will be difficult but might be more difficult later.'
Ania took a deep breath. It would be a big change, she thought to herself. She could understand it, but Maria would not. Maria knew a little about her country, and she knew a little about Croatia; Ania having made a point of telling her about it and showing her pictures. She wanted her to be familiar and to know that although she lived here she really belonged somewhere else.
The session continued with Ania saying more about the area she lived in, and about some of the places that she remembered visiting. Ania also had some

photos with her that she took out. At that point Maria decided that they were more interesting than her colouring book and helped by taking the photos from Ania and giving them to Debbie as Ania described what they were. Debbie listened, not saying much other than to remark on how she felt looking at the photos, and empathising with Ania's increasing enthusiasm for the places.

'Yes, you like to be here but your home is there.' Debbie was responding to a comment Ania had made about feeling she did not belong in England, though was grateful for being there.

'Yes, I like to be here, we like to be here, don't we, Masza?' She turned to look at her daughter, who was nodding enthusiastically, 'but one day we must go back to these places ...' Go back. She somehow wanted to go forward. She understood the English meaning of going back, but she could not go back, things had changed. Things were and would be different. It was another part of the uncertainty of her future. But she knew it would be OK, she would make it good. There were good people in her family, though she was aware that not everyone had indicated in their letters that they accepted Maria, or herself as one of the 'raped women' in her country.

After the session was over Debbie found herself pondering on Ania's future and wondering what would be for the best. She knew that Ania had a difficult decision to make although it seemed that she had made her decision; it was more that she needed reassurance that she was making the right one. Who could really offer that reassurance? She wanted Ania to feel that it was her decision, but she knew that she was likely to be influenced by the people she talked to, particularly at the social group she now attended.

She was pleased to have met Maria. She looked at Maria's picture and smiled. It was actually a really colourful picture, and the big smiles that she had drawn on her and Ania's faces made Debbie smile too. A thought cut into her mind as she looked at it and she felt the tears welling up in her own eyes. She was back in the last session with Ania. She had this picture because of the terrible events that had occurred, because of Ania being raped. It was one of those moments when horror and beauty clashed, when there was no way of bringing them together, all that could be done was to acknowledge the presence of both, and celebrate Maria as a little girl in the world facing her own uncertain future, a little girl who liked to draw and to colour ...

* * *

Ania sat at home that evening. Her thoughts were very much alive to her. Maria was in bed – she was glad that she slept so peacefully although sometimes she felt she would have been glad if Maria disturbed her in the evening. It helped to break her chain of thoughts.

She had kept in contact with friends and family in Croatia and she had a good idea of how things now were. She knew she had to go back one day to relatives in Croatia – at least to begin with. There was nothing really left for her in Bosnia, just painful memories that seemed to wipe out the good memories of what she had experienced before . . .

She knew how many women who had been raped sought abortions, and many who gave birth placed the children in orphanages. She had decided to have her child. She really did not know why, so many thoughts and feelings had been present for her. It had not felt right for her to have an abortion, even though she understood why other women had made that choice. Her religious beliefs had played a part in the decision. But having given birth to Maria, she knew she could not have handed her over to an orphanage. She was glad to be in England where she was simply a single mother – a mother with a history that few knew, but she was not treated differently because she had been one of the thousands of 'raped women' who she understood were being shunned within Bosnian society.

It was good to be mixing with people from her own country. Just hearing her own language – yes, she had met up with other people from Bosnia since being in England, but there was something about being amongst a *group* of people. It had touched something deep in her, and it had left her feeling sad as well, sad for the country and for the people. Next week there was going to be some music and traditional dances. She was looking forward to that. They were so important to her culture and whilst she knew that perhaps they meant more to generations before her, they had always been special for her.

It was getting late and she knew she must try to get some sleep. The tablets the doctor had prescribed to her did help, but not every night. She got up, took a look around her living room, turned off the light and closed the door. She could hear the sound of the traffic outside as she walked up the small hallway towards her bedroom, stopping only to gently push open the door to Maria's room. All was quiet, she could hear her breathing as she walked over to the bed, and leaning over gently kissed her on the forehead. There was a slight stir. She tucked the sheet up under her chin. Love and pain, hope and sadness. She turned and left the room, there were tears in her eyes . . .

* * *

Debbie was sitting at home and had picked up an article that she had been emailed. It was timely, and it was not easy reading. Although it was about Bosnia; rape, mutilation and torture had a high incidence by all sides in civil and inter-country wars. She thought about the impact of rape on the women and their children, how devastating it is in so many ways, having far-reaching personal, familial and social consequences. The article was written in 2002. The source was the Institute for War and Peace Reporting, Balkans.[2]

---

[2] This article is reprinted here with the intention to inform the reader and to provide real background to the situation that has developed in Bosnia with regard to raped women and their children. Belma Becirbasic and Dzenana Secic are journalists with *Start* magazine in Sarajevo. They were awarded the Amnesty International Global Award for Human Rights Journalism 2003 for this piece of investigative journalism.

Invisible casualties of war

Bosnia's raped women are being shunned by a society that refuses to see them as victims

By Belma Becirbasic and Dzenana Secic, Sarajevo

Nine-year-old Edin is one of thousands of children in Bosnia growing up without a father. But while others have a grave to visit, or photographs to treasure, Edin has neither. His mother Safeta has one single, terrible memory of his father. 'He lit a candle or a lighter and made his choice,' she said. 'He was a Serb from Zemun. Even 20 years from now I'd recognize him.'

Safeta is a 'raped woman', to use a label which became commonplace for women who fell victim to systematic sexual abuse in the first year of the Bosnian war. Edin's father is the man who raped her. Today, these women are the invisible casualties of the war, overlooked and often shunned. The fate of their children is even more tragic. Edin is one of a tiny minority who live with their birth mothers – many of the other women abandoned their babies, or even murdered them. In the summer of 1992, chilling reports of mass deportations from eastern Bosnia and detention camps in north-west Bosnia were accompanied by accounts of mass rape. There were even rumours of a plan to impregnate thousands of non-Serb women to fuel ethnic hatred. The exact numbers of women raped will never be known, not least since some of the victims were later murdered. The highest estimate, delivered to a European Union commission in Brussels in February 1993, was 50 000.

Behind the statistics were women like Safeta, detained for three days in an abandoned house outside Zvornik, north-east Bosnia. There, she was raped by one of a group of soldiers and volunteers from Serbia. Two 17-year-old girls were detained with her. 'One of them, Amra, was raped by 13 men,' she said. Safeta, then 29, was luckier – she was raped only once. Today, Safeta and Edin live together in a small house in Zivince, outside Tuzla. The former works at the Vive Zena womens' centre in Tuzla, which provides counselling for rape victims and includes some raped women among its staff. Now 40, she talks openly about her experiences, turning away only occasionally. But she is unusual. Shame and ostracisim drive many women to conceal their ordeals, another reason a definitive estimate has been so difficult to establish. Safeta's story has an uplifting ending, but it sheds light on the tragic experiences of the many women. Many raped women were deliberately kept in detention until it was too late for them to get an abortion. Safeta was six months pregnant by the time she arrived in Tuzla, and no one would perform the operation at that late stage. Edin was born on April 14 1993. Unable to prevent his birth, his mother refused to even look at him, claiming she would strangle him. Edin was deposited in a Tuzla orphanage, and Safeta began her life as a refugee in Zivince.

Teufika Ibrahimefendic, a clinical psychologist at the Vive Zena centre, where Safeta works, said, 'It is the women who have kept their ordeal a secret for the last ten years who concern psychiatrists the most. They conceal it to try and protect themselves, but this creates an intolerable pressure. I once heard a woman describe how every time she remembers being raped, she stands under a cold shower until she freezes.'

The Hague tribunal has recognised that rape was used as a systematic weapon of ethnic cleansing in Bosnia, making it indictable as a war crime. Rape formed part of the case against the three-member Foca group, sentenced to a total of 60 years in prison for crimes against humanity committed in eastern Bosnia in the early Nineties. Ante Furundzija, the commander of a special Bosnian Croat unit in central Bosnia was charged with watching the rape of a Bosnian woman, not intervening and not punishing the rapists. Proceedings against Hazim Delic in connection with the Celebici prison camp also confirmed rape as a war crime.

But regardless of international law, raped women are still not recognized as victims within Bosnia. At best, they are regarded as tarnished, at worst as 'fallen women' who somehow invited their own misfortune. For years, Safeta says she endured the whispers and pointing fingers of other women in Zivince. The taboo around rape even extended to her family. Her mother, sister and brother-in-law were supportive, but not her father or younger brother. 'My father never asked me what had happened or where my child was,' she said.

Safeta remained in Bosnia throughout her pregnancy, but many women who had been raped in prison camps in north-west Bosnia were evacuated to third countries via Croatia. Director of the Zagreb Centre for Women Victims of War, CWVW, Nela Pamukovic, recalled two pregnant raped women who took refuge with her organisation, 'One of them kept her baby and left for the US with her parents. The other threw her newly-born child into the Sava river. She was charged with infanticide, but did not stand trial after doctors diagnosed diminished responsibility.'

Like Safeta, many women rejected their babies immediately after giving birth. In Zagreb, most deliveries took place at the Petrovo maternity hospital. From there, according to CWVW and the Zagreb Caritas office, unwanted babies were taken to the Vladimir Nazor orphanage or the Goljak centre for children with special needs. At this point, it becomes difficult to keep track of the babies. Records were kept of all children admitted, but staff had no way of knowing which babies were the offspring of raped mothers, not least because some women didn't tell anyone they had been raped.

Moreover, the aftermath of war in Croatia and the raging conflict in Bosnia made tracking the children even harder. 'We didn't keep track of any of the children who came to us in that period,' said a hospital source who did not want to be named. 'Our priority was to provide them with care, regardless of where they came from.'

Zagreb Caritas received around 150 raped women, of whom around 60 per cent were pregnant. Director Jelena Brajsa remembers the first 15 pregnant women who arrived in 1993. All had been repeatedly raped. After delivery, four babies were transferred to Obrenovo for medical treatment, two mothers kept their babies and the remaining nine were collected by the Bosnian embassy and Red Cross and later returned to Bosnia. There, two were taken by their families, two were adopted and the remainder placed in institutions.

In general, the babies suffered from the stigma of the crime which had created them. 'I once attended a meeting of the Association of Bosnian Women in Zagreb, which is now defunct,' said Brajsa. 'They discussed the fate of babies of raped women and there was a general consensus that these children should be taken as far away from Bosnia as possible.'

A doctor at the Goljak centre for children with special needs recalls how nine children of raped women were admitted to the centre in 1995. He even considered adopting one of the children. 'One little boy was very sweet and I spent a lot of time with him. However, my wife, who is Bosnian herself, wouldn't even consider adoption. People have something against these children, even though they are not to blame for any of this.' He does not know where the children went after they left the centre.

Six months after leaving her son in a Tuzla orphanage, Safeta set out to find him. Thoughts of the baby had been haunting her. 'I couldn't sleep for four months. After six months it became unbearable. If I hadn't found him when I did, I probably wouldn't be alive now,' she said. A social worker told Safeta that her son had been admitted to hospital. Edin was suffering from malnutrition and had chewed his fingers to the bone. When she found him, she held him silently for 20 minutes. 'I could see that he looked like me and that he was healthy. I don't know how I made it home that day,' she recalled.

Although neither she nor Edin ever left Bosnia, Safeta was still fortunate to find her son. Orphanages and hospitals were overloaded and other women who underwent a change of heart may not have been so lucky. 'In 1993 alone, we admitted 700 children and the capacity of the orphanage was only 110,' said Advija Hercegovac of the Vojo Peric orphanage in Tuzla. 'It is possible that many of those were the babies of raped women, but there was chaos at the time and we had more important tasks than keeping detailed records.' Children who were later adopted were subject to the usual rules protecting their identities and those of their adoptive parents. Finding Edin was not the end of the story for Safeta. He remained in the orphanage for another seven years, while his mother summoned up the courage and the means to bring him home. Raped women who kept their babies are a tiny minority, according to Fadila Memisevic of the Association for the Threatened Peoples of Bosnia. Many more may have wanted to do so, but the pressures they were placed under were intolerable.

Mirha Pojskic of Medica, an NGO in Zenica which focuses on helping traumatised women, recalls the case of one woman who was raped close to the border with Serbia. Even though she was a Bosniak, the woman fled to Serbia where she adopted a Serbian name. Unable to tell even her closest family about her rape and pregnancy, the woman gave birth and kept her child for a year. Finally, with no money or family support, she left him in a Serbian orphanage. The orphanage discovered that the baby was a Bosnian citizen and insisted that she remove him.

She then took her son to her own parents in Sarajevo, but they refused to accept him. He, in turn, developed a constant fear that his mother would abandon him. After some months, Pojskic received a letter from the Sarajevo social services saying the woman wanted Medica to take in her baby, because she could no longer feed him. 'I begged the welfare people in Sarajevo to find the woman a job so she could her support her child, but they did nothing,' she said.

Another woman approached Medica after being raped in Brcko. She was accompanied by her mother, who kept insisting the pregnancy was her daughter's own fault. In the end, this woman did manage to keep her child. After a period of living alone and drinking heavily, Safeta began to stitch her life back together. She found a job, bought a piece of land and started building a house. She visited her son regularly and was driven by a vision of living with him under the same roof. 'That was what I lived for, the moment when darkness would turn into light. And if people disapproved, I couldn't care less,' she said.

At the beginning of this year, Pojskic launched a campaign to obtain civilian war victim status for women who were raped. This status, granted by the ministry for human rights and refugees, has a number of benefits attached. 'By entitling them to health insurance and other benefits granted to victims of war, by helping them to find jobs, we hope that women will finally come forward and admit they were raped. We may then find out how many women were victims of this crime,' she said. Currently, only former camp detainees are recognised as civilian victims. It is hoped that by extending this status to raped women, they will be de-stigmatised. Official recognition of their trauma may finally dispel the notion – most prevalent in small towns and villages – that they were in some way responsible for what happened to them. Today, Safeta proudly shows off photos of her son. With blue eyes and light brown hair, he takes after her. Traces of the ordeal mother and son have endured can be seen in a certain reserve between them. 'Sometimes I feel an urge to hug him, to kiss him all over, but I only ever kiss him at night, while he is asleep,' she said. Edin too is discreet. Hidden behind a curtain, he likes to stand at the window and wait for his mother to arrive home from work. He has never asked about his father.

Points for discussion

- Evaluate Debbie's person-centred responses in this session. Which were most significant, and why?
- Would you have responded differently to Maria being brought to the session?
- Evaluate the significance of having Maria at the session. What may have changed for the therapeutic relationship in future sessions because of her attendance in that session, assuming she does not attend again?
- What are your feelings at the end of the session, and after reading the article above? How might reading this affect your way of being with Ania if you were her counsellor?
- What might you take to supervision from this session?
- Write notes for this session.

CHAPTER 7

Supervision session 2: Sympathy, empathy, healing and 'not for healing'

Rob listened to what Debbie was saying with a particular intensity and focus. Debbie was describing the session in which Ania had talked about what had happened to her and her brother. It was not something to be able to listen to and not be affected by. He was concerned for his supervisee. What effect was it having on her? What would she need from the supervision session to help her continue to be present for her client? There may be issues to work through, she may simply need to tell the story herself, talk it through, make sense of her own feelings and thoughts, her own very human reactions to the atrocities that her client had experienced and which were now experiences communicated to Debbie.

'What do you say?' Debbie paused. 'I really felt affected, and thank God I was, I mean, when I stop being affected is the day to quit and do something else.' She was shaking her head.

'Yeah, we have to be affected, it's part of what we offer.'

'And the thought I was left with was that it didn't matter how much it affected me, however intense any feelings I may have, they are still as nothing compared to those of Ania.'

'I want to acknowledge that and I want to say, don't underestimate the intensity of the impact on you, Debbie.'

'I know, but in a way it doesn't matter, and I know it does. I know it does.' Debbie paused. She was surprised and not surprised about the intensity of the feelings that were becoming present in her as she talked about the session, about what Ania had said, and gave herself time to re-live the impact it had, and continued to have on her. 'It would be so easy to sympathise.'

Rob nodded, 'yes, and you know, sometimes I wonder whether that is what is needed.'

Debbie looked at him. 'Even though we are supposed to empathise, not sympathise?'

'Can we avoid conveying sympathy? Can we really? We may not use the words, but the look in our eyes, the expression on our faces when someone describes some painful or tragic episode? What's an empathic expression on your face? How do you look empathic, Debbie?'

Debbie thought about it. 'I don't know. I guess you can mirror your client's expression.'

'Hmm, but I think we communicate sympathy too through facial expression and so long as we do not replace empathy with sympathy, I do not see that this human reaction is unhelpful for a client, particularly when they witness us being affected by something that perhaps they struggle to accept is significant enough for them to acknowledge the effect on them.' Rob took a deep breath. He knew he'd stepped away from where Debbie was focused. It was his issue, he knew that, but he struggled with this notion that he often came across in some areas of the counselling world where empathy was seen as 'good' and sympathy almost as something 'bad'.

'You mean the look that says, "how terrible", though without the words?'

'Can we control our facial expression that much when we are touched, affected by a client's experience? And what happens to our congruence once we try to contain or alter a natural and spontaneous and very human reaction?'

Whilst it is true that empathy is encouraged and sympathy is frowned upon, or so it seems in the counselling world, the person-centred counsellor who is affected by the distress of another is going to communicate sympathy through facial expression and the look in their eyes. And they will communicate compassion and maybe horror. Yes, a counsellor isn't going to say 'poor thing', but how many times will counsellors say in supervision – 'I feel so much for her', 'how can anyone keep going after that' – or just simply sit shaking their heads at the awesome challenges that clients have faced and found ways to come through. I believe that feelings of sympathy – sorrow that someone has had to go through an experience – is a valid human reaction. Yes, it is unlikely to be verbalised in a session, but it is going to be felt. And maybe, when it is felt, then there will be times when congruence demands that it be voiced.

Sometimes sympathy may be with the person, sometimes with the situation. I've heard myself say to clients, when they have described a situation and we have wrestled with it, and maybe they are feeling hopeless; 'it's a bugger, isn't it?' Is this sympathy? I'm not saying, 'you poor thing, how awful for you.' But maybe my responding is close to sympathy, maybe situational sympathy rather than personal sympathy.

At other times the client will see sympathy in the counsellor's eyes. I know if I have said something expressive of pain and distress, I would want to see my counsellor touched and affected. Yes, I would want to see a sympathetic reaction, and a compassionate reaction, as well as a constant striving to show me that they are hearing and appreciating what it is I am experiencing and wanting to have heard. We talk a lot of clients feeling heard, but clients also want what they are experiencing to be felt by their counsellor. I do not want to feel adrift on a turbulent ocean of my own experiencing, although it may feel that way at times. I want someone else to know how damned turbulent it is, what it feels like trying to stay afloat. And I want them to offer a safe and secure place where I can feel some relief from the turbulence, or should I say, I want them to be with me in a way that might enable me to find that place in myself.

'We talked last time about being human, about what we have to offer is ourselves, and I remember talking about the heart, about heartfelt responses – or did I? I know the idea of heartfelt responding is something that has been in my own thoughts recently.'

'I think you did, I know the heart certainly came up as a theme.' Rob couldn't recall exactly what had been said.

'And now Ania is trying to decide whether to stay here or return home – at least, return to Croatia, to family, and rebuild her life over there, as much I think for Maria as herself.'

'Hmm. Whether to go back.'

'It's one of those "who knows what's best?" decisions, isn't it? So long as she can make her own decision.'

'Internal locus of evaluation?'

Debbie nodded. 'It's such an important decision, and I think she knows deep down what she needs to do, or is it need, or is it want?'

Rogers wrote of the importance of developing an internal locus of evaluation. He described this, in the context of creativity, in the following terms. 'Perhaps the most fundamental condition of creativity is that the source or locus of evaluative judgement is internal. The value of his product is, for the creative person, established not by the praise or criticism of others, but by himself. Have I created something satisfying to *me*? Does it express a part of me – my feeling or my thought, my pain or my ecstasy?' (Rogers, 1967, p. 354).

How is this arrived at? What moves the person from an external to an internal locus of evaluation? Merry suggests the following: 'The counsellor's attendance to non-judgemental, empathic understanding of the client's world of inner experiencing amounts, for the client, to an experience of unconditional positive regard. The counselling relationship provides, in essence, a corrective experience where the perception of authentic unconditional positive regard leads to an increase in positive self-regard. Admitting into awareness previously denied or distorted experiencing results in a reorganisation of the self-concept, the self-concept becomes increasingly congruent with experience, and the locus of evaluation tends to become internal rather than external' (Merry, 2002, pp. 56–7).

'How are you with that, with being with her in that process, given how important it is to be offering the core conditions to encourage movement towards a greater sense of internal evaluation?'

'I feel OK with it. I have had my congruence challenged at times, and it has been challenging for me. But it feels as though there is greater and maybe deeper connection now. I do believe I am offering unconditional positive regard, and it is genuine and heartfelt. And I feel my empathy is there, though the depth of pain and distress is over my horizon of experiencing, as it often is with my clients as you know. It feels as though my horizon has expanded through my work in this area. I can appreciate far more the depths of distress people can feel, how disorganised they can feel inside as a result of their experiences. But there is always a new twist.' Debbie shook her head. Yes, her work with clients who were victims of warfare did push her – not that they did personally though sometimes they did, but it was what they brought into the sessions. 'I guess everyone says it, but I think this really is one of the most difficult areas to work in. It's the mix of pain, and horror, and inhumanity as well.'

'Hmm.' Rob could sense that Debbie had not finished and he did not want to interrupt her flow.

'It's the inhumanity that's hardest to get your head around.'

Rob guessed that was what was going to be acknowledged and it was another reason why he had not responded. He wanted Debbie to acknowledge it herself.

'Yes, inhumanity, atrocity, readiness of a human-being to inflict pain on another.'

'And I know it doesn't just happen in war, Rob, people get abducted, horrible things happen, but there is something about the chaos of warfare as well. It didn't used to be like that – well that's my fantasy. Two armies would fight it out. Now, well, it seems to be ordinary people that bear the brunt of it, all the time, and not just in war.'

'That really affects you, Debbie, how ordinary people bear the brunt of it.'

'I see the pain, Rob', there were tears in Debbie's eyes and her voice was breaking up, 'I see it, I hear it, I am filled with it, and however bad it gets for me, it is still as nothing compared to what they go through, nothing.' Sadness and anger overtook her, pain and outrage ripped into her heart. She buried her face in her hands. The build up had reached bursting point, it did from time to time.

'The utter, utter awfulness of it.' Rob reached over to Debbie and rubbed her shoulder.

'People, ordinary people, it's always ordinary people, their lives torn apart, often their bodies too.'

Rob continued to rub.

'Thanks.' She had taken hold of his wrist. 'Thanks.' She felt the emotion subsiding. 'I guess today was another day for it to burst out.'

'Yeah.'

'Ooohh.' She swallowed and took a tissue, drying her eyes and her face.

'You keep going back in there, Debbie, I admire you, it takes courage, you know.'

'I keep telling Ania she's courageous, she won't believe me.'

'Then you're as bad as each other! It's not an easy thing to own, but even when you can't own it, it's important to hear it, so long as the client is left feeling that they aren't being expected to feel courageous.'

'Ania can own being proud, but not courageous. Maybe one day. Maybe. But you don't have to own it to be it.'

'No, no you don't.'

Debbie was thinking of Ania and her situation. 'If she feels that need to return then I hope that is what she will do, and I hope that if she does do that her need will also be a want. She is a strong, courageous woman, Rob, she's survived, she is surviving, and Maria is delightful. I guess for me it is more a case of "when" she decides to return, I don't think there's any question that she will return.' The thought was with Debbie that she hoped that the counselling would help prepare her for that big step. 'I just hope I can play a part in helping her move forward, Rob. If I can feel that I've contributed to helping her to find that something inside herself to move into her future and, I suppose, make good of it, and not feel so affected by what she has experienced . . .' She paused. 'But then, well, I can't take the past away from her or from anyone.' She took a deep breath.

'No, we can't take away the past, only offer the therapeutic conditions in the hope – well, more the belief – that by so doing that person will be enabled to become how they want to be.' He paused, trying to find the right words as he wasn't sure he had expressed himself as he had wanted. 'It's hard to put into words, sometimes.'

'Sometimes it feels like we are patching people up – emotionally, psychologically, perhaps spiritually, before sending them back out. Some scars will maybe never heal, though.' Debbie was thinking of the experiences that Ania would always have with her.

'We must hope that their structure of self is re-organised through the experience of the therapeutic relationship such that they can experience greater wholeness, greater integration, greater self-awareness, greater congruence, but we cannot remove scars. We may provide the therapeutic relationship that is the healing environment, but we are not the healer. The clients self heal. We simply help that capacity for self-healing.'

'And people don't always want to heal, of course.'

Mearns, as mentioned earlier (Mearns and Thorne, 2000, pp. 114–16), has described 'growthful' and 'not-for growth' configurations within the self. It is not unreasonable to accept that there may also be 'healing' and 'not for healing' configurations. A person may be carrying a strong sense of self invested in being wounded in some way, in some part of their structure of self. The need to maintain that identity may override any internal process seeking to bring about healing. The offering of the therapeutic relationship should enable the client to begin to acknowledge and engage with the 'woundedness' in such a way as to begin the process of healing, but the 'not for healing' configuration if present will work against this.

The outcome will be dependent on the quality of the therapeutic relationship which will be linked to the therapist's capacity to offer and communicate the core conditions, the client's ability to receive the responses of the counsellor, and the degree to which the client has invested their self-concept in the 'not for healing' configuration where it is present.

The challenge is for the counsellor to offer the core conditions to the 'not for healing' part, to ensure that it is heard and understood, that it can be deserving of warmth and caring, unconditionally. Then gradually the client may begin to risk moving their identity a little from that configuration into another part, or a new part may emerge carrying a stronger healing imperative, or maybe the 'not for healing' part itself may change, taking the person's sense of self with it to contribute to the formation of a new self-concept.

'Depends I suppose how we define "healing".' Rob paused. 'We seem to be heading into a rather philosophical discussion here. I just wanted to acknowledge that and question whether that is how you want to use the time.'

Debbie thought for a moment. Her thoughts were back with Ania. 'Somehow I feel uncomfortable. Yes, to have a philosophical discussion in the context of what Ania has experienced does not feel right. Thank you for saying that. I do want to stay with those feelings that are present for me. She told me how important it was for her to tell me about what happened, she wanted me to hear. I am wanting to honour that, Rob.' Debbie felt her own emotions rising to the surface, and her own eyes watering. 'She told me. I know it could have been any counsellor, probably, but it was me.'

'That sense of *you* having been told, that it was important for *you* to hear.'

Debbie nodded. She looked down. 'Me as a counsellor, but also me as a woman.'

'As a counsellor, as a woman.'

Debbie nodded. 'And maybe important for her to tell someone from outside of her country as well.'

'Sure. All very important.' Rob appreciated the seriousness and the importance of what was now being said. Clients needed to tell their stories, and sometimes they needed to take a lot of time before they could begin to, sometimes it happened sooner. Some took their time and had to repeat it, others did not need it heard more than once. Ania had needed Debbie to hear her story. Rob was aware that the story would be told not just in words, but in thoughts and feelings, in emotion, in presence, through the way of being of the client as they sought to communicate what they needed to say, what they needed to hear themselves say, how they needed to be, and how they needed the other person – the counsellor – to receive what they were communicating.

'I believe I have heard her, but I think there is more of her to be communicated to me, Rob. There was emotion and pain, and hurt, and terror, but it was one part of one session. She wanted to tell me, but maybe for a logical reason. I think there is an emotional need as well, and I don't think that side has really emerged yet, not with me. She hasn't let go or let it go.'

'And maybe she will, and maybe she won't. She will work with it as she will. But your sense is that there will be, that there is, more to emerge.'

'Of course, I don't know what has happened previously. Maybe she has. Maybe, maybe not. I don't know. I don't believe in rigid timescales on any of this.'

'Everyone's an individual. We accept them, their process, the parts of them that emerge, that are shown to us, and we stay with them, beside them.'

'I need to be able to be with her, to listen, to listen with my being not just my ears.'

Rob nodded.

'And I may be on the phone to you if it feels overwhelming.'

'Please do. It can be tempting not to . . .'

'. . . I'm not the "heroic counsellor" type who can stand and take it all. I'm a human-being like anyone else who is perfectly capable of being overwhelmed. I have to be able to be fully present not just for Ania, but for my other clients as well.'

'And for yourself in your own life.'

Debbie smiled wryly. 'Yes.' She paused. 'It puts your own life into perspective though.'

* * *

Over the next few weeks, Ania continued to attend the counselling sessions. She talked about her thoughts for the future, the family group, Maria, and brought more photos in of her past and of her country. It seemed to Debbie that she was in a sense showing signs of integrating her experience more fully into her awareness and whilst there was emotional upset during the sessions, it seemed as though it was controlled. Debbie was aware of some misgivings, wondering whether the control would last, whether a further release was necessary. However, she trusted implicitly Ania's need to be how she was. She needed to talk in the way that she was and for Debbie there was an acceptance of this. She listened, she stayed with her as she talked of her life. And yet . . . somehow, there was a depth of emotion that was not present, a sense that there was something being held back, or which simply was not finding a way through into expression.

As a person-centred counsellor, Debbie well recognised the need for her clients to be allowed to be how they needed to be. She trusted the presence of the actualising tendency, that this essential drive within the person would be seeking to enable them to be in a way that was fulfilling to them. Debbie could see, as well, how so much of Ania's positive view of life was being lived through her relationship with Maria. She wondered how Ania would be in the future when Maria was at school every day, but then, maybe they would be in Croatia by then and, well, things would be as they would be. She had to be philosophical. Ania's prime identity was very much as a mother. A whole system of thoughts, feelings and behaviours had clearly developed around this and contributed to what might be termed as a 'configurational state'. This was where, if you like, the actualising tendency had its strongest focus, that was what she was growing into, and it was wonderful to see, and yet . . .

At her next supervision session, Debbie discussed her sense that there was something else, some other aspect or aspects of Ania that were not finding expression. How much they were present to Ania's awareness, she did not know. But Ania had reported that her sleep had become more disturbed and that she was feeling generally more unsettled, restless in herself, more affected by the memories at times. It was as though the better times were getting better but the painful times were becoming more intense. Ania's social worker, Gina, had been on the phone, concerned that counselling was making Ania worse. Debbie had to explain that whilst this might be the case, in the greater process it was likely that it was a phase to be worked through. She did not go into great detail, but simply pointed out that Ania had been exposed to extremely difficult experiences and that they may not all emerge straight away. She indicated that clients could not be hurried, that they had to be trusted. She would continue to work with Ania, giving her the space that she needed and the therapeutic experience that would help her to allow anything that needed to be dealt with to emerge into awareness and into the therapeutic relationship, when the time was right.

Debbie had also dropped a note to Ania's GP. It had been an idea that had been suggested by Gina that Ania had brought to Debbie. In this Debbie confirmed that the counselling continued, the issues that were being addressed, that it was an on-going process, that Ania found the sleeping tablets helpful although at present her sleep was more disturbed. Ania had seen and agreed with the letter.

Throughout this period Ania was aware in herself that she was feeling at times stronger and yet at other times more fragile. The evenings were still difficult but she had made friends through the family group and she talked some evenings with some of the other mothers. She was also writing letters to family and seeking advice about returning within the next 18 months. But she could not get the memories out of her head, and not just out of her head. Out of her body, too. She would be compulsive in her washing. She did not think of it that way, but she would take much longer than she used to, standing in the shower and losing all track of time. She would wash her genital area again and again at night and in the mornings, thinking that she might not be clean enough. She had not spoken of this to Debbie or to Gina. And she was going out less. She went to the counselling, she went to the family group, she saw Gina at home, she went shopping and occasionally took Maria to the park, but not as much as she had in the past.

CHAPTER 8

Counselling session 11: bad dreams and more emotional release

Ania had experienced a difficult week, and she felt quite drained. Her nights had
become very disturbed, dreams that made no sense to her, faces of men she did
not know and yet she did. There was a familiarity but who were they? She'd
wake up feeling real fear, sweating, the bed covers in a tangle. On one occasion
she had woken Maria by her shouting in the dream, and she had woken to
find Maria by the bed looking anxious. It was this that had made Ania realise
she needed to say something to Debbie today. She had hugged Maria, tried to
reassure her that she was OK, and had let Maria stay in bed with her the rest
of that night.

'So, how do you want to use our time today, Ania?'

Ania looked down. Her heart was thumping and she felt strangely numb in her
arms and legs. 'I-I'm not sure. It's been difficult.' She was still looking down.

'Difficult?'

Ania nodded. 'I-I haven't been sleeping too good.'

'Mhmm, sleep's got bad.'

'I have these dreams, you call them nightmares, I think?'

'Mhmm, yes, scary dreams, yes?'

'Terrible dreams, but I don't know what I dream, but I see faces and I am frightened, so frightened, and I feel awful when I wake up, just awful.'

'Faces that frighten you in your dreams?'

Ania nodded. They were present now as she spoke. Men with awful expressions
on their faces. 'I-I don't know who they are, but I wake up so frightened,
Debbie.' She told her about Maria waking up and coming to her in the night.
'I don't want to worry her, she was so frightened, I could see it in her eyes. But
what was it, Debbie? I do not understand. I have enough nightmares that I do
understand, I don't need more.'

'I don't know, Ania, but I do hear how you feel you don't need more nightmares.'

The session continued with Ania saying more about the dreams, the faces,
the feelings, but she could not say anything else. It upset her greatly and
most of the session then became focused once more on the events that she

remembered, with more emotional release. Debbie maintained her empathy and unconditional positive regard, feeling for Ania as the feelings emerged. To Debbie the tone of her upset seemed different, seemed somehow more convulsive, she couldn't think of another word.

'I feel very shaky, Debbie, and I must be strong for Maria. I cannot let her see me like this.'

'That's really important for you, Ania, being strong for Maria.'

'I have to be, but I am not sure how it will be when I am like this.'

'That worries you.'

'It does, very much. I-I wish I . . . , oh, I can cope with the memories, I have coped, I do cope, but this feels like something I do not know. I do not know how to deal with what I do not know. Do people have dreams like this, Debbie? Is this what happens?'

'People do have dreams.' Debbie was very careful in what she said, not wanting to suggest to Ania that there might be other memories that she had not recovered. But for Debbie it was feeling increasingly like that, and it made sense for her as to why she had been feeling there was something else. 'And it leaves you feeling there is something you do not know.'

The counsellor needs to be careful when clients are talking about memories, or things they sense but do not know. In general, if a client is feeling this disturbed by dreams then the 'dreams' are carrying some memory that has not yet been fully brought into awareness. But the person-centred counsellor cannot directly encourage this process, suggest that this is the case, or try and interpret what is being dreamed. All must proceed at its own pace. The counsellor can reassure, empathise, convey warmth and support. They can make themselves available for the client should something emerge into awareness, perhaps ensuring the client knows they can call them if they need to, and when they would be available for this, but not in a way to alarm the client. For example, 'If you feel it is too much, and you want to call, please do. I can be available between . . . At any other time, leave a message and I'll get back to you as soon as I can.'

'Yes, I do not know, and I cannot deal with it. And I cannot accept it, it doesn't feel right. How can I know something but not know what it is, Debbie? I cannot accept that. I try to cope, I do cope, I have been coping. So many bad things, but I cope. But I cannot accept the nightmares.'

'You cannot accept knowing something that you do not know, or the bad things that have happened?'

'I do not accept them. Yes, bad things happened, Debbie, things I will not accept, things that were not right. But people were treated worse than me. It just seemed that things were getting better, and going to the family group has been really good, and now . . . , now I feel like I cannot cope.'

Debbie nodded, 'yes, that is how it feels when these awful nightmares upset you. You feel you cannot cope.'

'But I must, I will.' Ania sniffed and took a tissue. 'I have to.'

'Mhmm.'

Ania blew her nose. 'Oh.' And then took a deep breath.

Time had passed and there was not much more time left in the session.

'How are you feeling now, Ania?'

'I will be OK. I am sure that the dreams will pass. Perhaps I should see the doctor. What do you think?'

'Do you think it would help?'

'I may be able to have something stronger to help me sleep.'

'Yes, you might.'

'I will see how I am this week and then decide.'

'Mhmm, see how you feel. And if you need to call, please do. I cannot guarantee how soon I can call you back if I am seeing clients.' Debbie went on to explain which days she was at the centre. Ania felt pleased about that although she did not think she would need to call. But she thanked Debbie.

The session drew to a close with Debbie again checking Ania was feeling OK to leave. She said that she was, and Debbie felt it was important for her to accept that. She sat down after the session to write her notes and wondered how the week was going to be for Ania, whether the dreams might bring further distress and other clearer memories that were currently unknown to her. She knew she had to be there for Ania without encouraging memories, or interpreting what she was experiencing as indicating anything in particular. She sensed, however, that the next session might be more intense, it seemed that the distress Ania was experiencing was increasing and was likely to be indicative that something was going to break into her awareness.

Counselling session 12: recovered memories – 'can I ever be clean?'

It was two days later, Gina had phoned. Ania was in a bad way, very distressed, saying she needed to talk to Debbie. Debbie had checked her diary and had agreed to see Ania the following day for an extra counselling session if that was what Ania wanted. It was. Ania arrived looking very pale, her eyes were dark, she had put on some make up but it did not disguise the change in her appearance.

'Ania, come in, please, sit down.' Debbie felt immediately concerned, yet did not want to say something that might direct Ania to any particular focus, and yet her concern felt as though it needed to be expressed and communicated.

Ania sat down. At first she looked down and then looked up, meeting Debbie's eyes briefly, and then looked away again. Debbie could see pain in Ania's eyes, pain and sadness, a kind of emptiness, and yet she also knew these were in part her interpretations. But she also knew something had happened, and whilst she trusted that her own facial expression would convey something of what she felt, she also felt that she needed to add a verbal response as well given that Ania had only looked at her so very briefly. Debbie responded. 'What's wrong?'

'I have remembered.' She said no more, but looked up again, straight at Debbie. It was a look that she would never forget. It was a look of horror.

'You have remembered.' Debbie kept her response simple and with a tone of voice that was a mixture of affirmation with a hint of questioning. She knew her face and eyes would still be expressing concern.

Ania nodded. Her body began to shake, seemingly uncontrollably, and Debbie wondered if she was about to fit.

'It is OK, it will pass.' Ania continued to look at Debbie.

Debbie leant forward and offered to hold Ania's hands. Ania took Debbie's hands in hers. Her grip was tight, and then it relaxed a little as the shaking began to ease.

'I thought I was only raped by the men who came to the house, who murdered Tomas, but it was not so.'

'You mean . . .'

'. . . there were others.'

'. . . other men raped you.' Debbie could feel a horrible sickening feeling deep down, low down, in her body. The room was suddenly very, very quiet. Debbie's senses were utterly alive, she could have heard the slightest sound, seen the slightest movement.

These moments of utter quiet occur in therapy. The counsellor must respect them and stay with them. The heightened sensitivity is an indicator of the importance of the material that is emerging. It can indicate material coming from depth. Working with recovered memories can be intense and requires concentration and focus. There can be dissociated parts (Bryant-Jefferies, 2003a; Warner 2000) which may emerge and which the client may be totally unaware of. It can be profoundly shocking and the client will need support to deal with the process of recovery as well as with the memories that have been recovered.

Ania nodded. 'Before I remembered the first soldiers coming and what happened, and then when I awoke and found . . .' she swallowed, 'my brother's hand. I did not know what had happened after the soldiers left. I did not know there were others.'

'You did not know that others had raped you?'

'No, but now I remember, and I remember that they had other women with them, and they raped them as well, and one of them was a young girl. I do not know her name – she was very young. I was tied down, I do not know how long it lasted, it was far worse than before. These men were different, brutal, they liked to hurt me.' Ania broke into another language, and tears poured down her face. Her body convulsed with sobs as she continued to talk in what Debbie assumed was her own tongue. It meant little to her, but she kept her focus and moved closer to hold Ania.

'Say it how you need to say it, Ania, say it in your own words.'

Ania continued to speak, her voice so full of pain and emotion. It was as though the emotion took over, the pain, and now the anger. She talked for some while, pausing now and then, the sobs and the convulsions continuing. It was some while before Ania began to speak again in English. 'The men in my dreams.' She cursed them in her own language, and then said what sounded to Debbie like a prayer. When she stopped she spoke again in English. 'I pray for those other women. I do not know what happened. I do not know. I remember the moaning and the screams, and I do not know how I got away, or what happened. I do not know. I remember it and then I still do not know what happened, and then I was at the hospital. And I do not understand how I had my brother's hand still with me. Perhaps they left but if they did, why did they leave me?' She shook her head. 'Why did they leave me? Why did I live?' The tears continued to fall, and Debbie was crying her own tears, hot and burning. She held Ania who held her back.

'It is a question difficult to answer, Ania, why did they leave you, why did you live?'

Ania's bodied tightened in a jerky manner. 'I am sorry, this happens, I do not understand.'

'Your body is still reacting to the trauma, Ania.'

'I do not think I will ever be clean.'

'Cannot imagine how you could ever feel clean.'

'I want to feel clean, but how can I? I was myself, Debbie, I was myself again and again, but I cannot be clean. I can never be clean. I CAN NEVER BE CLEAN!' Her voice increased in volume into a wail before she collapsed weakly into Debbie's arms once more, crying uncontrollably.

Debbie rubbed Ania's back gently but in a way that she hoped would communicate reassurance. The crying continued for some while, with no words passing between them. Debbie occasionally murmured reassuring sounds as Ania's tears and sobs began to ease. 'I thought it was bad but now,' her breath came in short bursts, 'now, now it is worse than ever.'

'Remembering these things, Ania, makes it feel so much worse.'

Ania swallowed. 'I have an appointment to see the doctor, but I wanted to see you first.'

'You want something to calm you down?'

'Yes, do you think that is right, I think I need something.'

'I'm sure it will be alright.'

'I don't think I can face this without something, and without you, and Gina – she's been wonderful. She has been so concerned, and I haven't told her, I wanted to tell you. I needed you to know first, Debbie.'

'I feel humbled, Ania, I really do. And I know that you are going to come through this. It is like bursting a boil.'

'What is a boil?'

'A swelling, a spot that is poisoned.'

'I understand. It is like letting the poison out?'

'Is that how it feels?'

'Yes, I think you are right, but it is horrible.'

'Yes, and it is good that it has come out, but so, so painful and distressing.'

'I feel as though I will go mad.'

Debbie nodded. 'Yes, like a madness.'

'But I knew, as soon as I . . . It was in a dream not last night but the night before. I began to remember. I did not want to remember, but it was like pictures were in my head that were not there before.'

Ania had relaxed her grip and Debbie eased hers and was easing back. She nodded, and moved around to the front of Ania, back to her seat, but continued to hold her hands.

'Oh Debbie, why are they such bastards, such animals!' Ania again cursed in her own language.

'Ania, it is good for you to speak in your own language. We sometimes need to use the right words that we sometimes cannot find in another language.'

'There is so much I want to say.'

'You can say it here. I will not understand your words but I am sure I will understand the feelings.'

Ania looked at Debbie, 'you think I should speak in my own words?'

'I think you should speak in whatever way that you feel you want and need to.'

Ania spoke again in her own language. Debbie listened to the sounds for that was all she was hearing, sounds that she could not attach specific meaning to, but the tone of voice conveyed feelings and expression. Ania's voice began softly, but with real hatred, venomous hatred as she spat the words out into the room, her voice increasing in volume though the pace of her speech remained slow and measured. Finally she stopped.

'I have to go home.'

Debbie responded, assuming, wrongly as it turned out, that Ania was referring to the counselling session. 'You wish to end the session early?'

'No, no, home, I have to return.'

'What has happened has made you realise even more that you have to go home?'

'Yes, yes, I must. I must. My people are there, the people who suffered as I did. I must be there, be with them. It is only right. I have been glad to be here. It has been important. It allowed me to meet you, but I must go back.'

Debbie adjusted to the sudden change of focus. 'Mhmm, you have to be with the people who suffered like you?'

Ania nodded. 'It is not easy for me to explain. We have talked a lot about it. But now I know. I must go to my relatives and then I must return to Bosnia, it is where I belong.'

'You sound very determined and sure, Ania.'

'I am. It was just now, when you said I should speak in my own words . . .'

Debbie was not sure she had quite put it like that, but let the comment go.

'... I realised that, yes, I did need to speak in my own words. There is a strength in my own words, and there is strength in me too. It gives me strength to speak like that.'

'Mhmm, to use your own words to convey your own thoughts and feelings.'

Ania nodded. 'I do not know when, but perhaps it must be sooner than I had thought. I am not sure.' She paused. 'Perhaps you think it is strange, having experienced what I have experienced, to want to go back.'

Debbie shook her head. 'No, Ania, I am not surprised. I am full of admiration and of wanting you to make decisions that are right for you. Perhaps I am surprised by the suddenness given your upset a short while ago.'

'Yes, and those feelings are close, Debbie, and they must remain close. I want to forget but I do not want to forget. We must never forget. But we must live on as well.'

'You seem to have changed so fast, Ania.'

'It is strange for me, too, but I must go home. It is like I have to face it there, face it where it happened. Do you understand?'

Debbie nodded slowly, 'I think so, but I cannot say I know what it feels like to be you as you say these things.'

'But you try, Debbie, and that means a lot to me.'

Debbie smiled and felt tears in her eyes and a lump in her throat. 'Yes, I try.'

Ania went quiet as her thoughts slid back into the experiences from her past that were now in her awareness. 'How can I feel clean, Debbie?'

Debbie did not hesitate in her response, which was congruent and utterly honest. 'I don't know, Ania, I wish I did . . . , I wish I did.'

'Washing does not help. It is inside me . . .' She closed her eyes as she spoke, feeling a rush of sickly revulsion in her stomach and a spontaneous tightening of her pelvic muscles. She shivered. 'It is inside my body, my bones, my muscles, and in my vagina . . . ,' she paused. 'And in my mouth, my throat. They forced that on me as well.'

Debbie instinctively felt herself close her eyes as she felt her own rush of revulsion. She opened them.

'Thank you for that reaction, Debbie, that is how it is.'

Debbie nodded.

'I need to heal my body. I need to wash away the poison. It is still there. I can feel it. I know it. I must find a way.'

'To cleanse and heal your body of the poison that is still there.'

'I have not let a man near me since I left Bosnia. I do not know if I can. I do not know.'

Debbie nodded again, 'you do not know if you can let a man near you.'

'He would have to be very gentle and understanding.' From looking sad Ania's face changed it became hard and angry. 'Those bastards robbed me of that too!'

Debbie took a deep breath. 'Robbed you of feeling you could be with a man.'

'I must be strong. In my anger is my strength, Debbie. I must not lose my anger.'

'Your anger sustains you?'

'And I cannot always be angry. I have to be a mother as well, and an angry mother will not be a good mother.'

'Mhmm, and it is important for you to be a good mother, not an angry mother.'

'Yes.' She paused. 'I pray, Debbie, every day. I pray for strength, I pray that I will find a way. I cannot pray for forgiveness, I do not forgive. But I pray that the terrible things that happened will not be repeated.' She paused. 'I do not understand how such things are allowed to happen, but there must be a reason, but I do not understand what it is.'

'Prayer is important to you, Ania, but why terrible things happen is a mystery.'

'Yes, that is right.'

Debbie had glanced at the clock, five minutes of the session left. 'We are soon out of time.'

'I am glad you could fit me in. I am very grateful.'

'Gina was very concerned, and that left me concerned, and I am glad you came. I am so sorry that you have discovered what you have discovered, but I do believe that poison must come out before the healing can begin.'

'I think I had begun to heal too quickly, perhaps. Maybe it made it more difficult for me to remember. But then, if I had remembered earlier, I do not know. I was not so strong. Perhaps I am stronger now.'

'Perhaps you are, Ania, perhaps now was the right time, is the right time.'

'Perhaps.' Ania paused, aware of the time and that she had to get back to Maria. Maria, she had not spoken of her hardly at all. 'I must go to Maria. Thank you, Debbie, thank you.' They were getting up and Ania came over and gave Debbie a hug, and kissed her on the cheek.

Points for discussion

- Were you anticipating the material in session 12 having read the sessions up to and including session 11? If so, why?
- Consider your own feelings as a result of reading the chapter. How will you process what you are left feeling and thinking?
- Evaluate Debbie's application of person-centred principles in the last two sessions.
- What were the key moments and how did the therapeutic relationship contribute to them?
- Is it reasonable that Ania seemed to switch so quickly in herself to the notion of returning 'home'? Explain this in terms of person-centred theory.
- Write notes for this session.

CHAPTER 9

Counselling session 13: tired of struggling, tired of living

'The memories remain with me, but I will survive them. I have survived when I could have been killed. Many were. I was perhaps fortunate, though at the time that would not have been my thinking. Now, well, I am alive, in England, with a lovely daughter.' Ania lapsed into silence. She was indeed fortunate, but so many had not been as fortunate as she. So many were dead, or perhaps more damaged by their ordeals as victims of the warfare in her land. It was not easy to accept her good fortune – if that was what it was – when so many had not survived.

'Mhmm, fortunate now but that would not have been how you would have described it before.'

Ania heard Debbie's response but it was in the distance. Her own thoughts and feelings were far more present for her. She sat staring ahead of her, but not really aware of anything beyond the heavy numbness that seemed to fill her whole being. Yes, she had survived, but why her? The young girl raped in her presence. She was sure she was dead. Was death a blessing? She didn't know. All she knew was that she was alive and others were not, and there was something deeply disturbing about that.

'It does not feel so right that I am alive.'

'Mhmm, given all that has happened, it does not feel so right to you to be alive.'

> Sometimes a comment such as this requires a simple, empathic response, at other times the empathic response may include a questioning tone. To know which is appropriate requires empathic sensitivity to the thoughts and feelings behind the words of the client. Sometimes it is therapeutically helpful to facilitate further exploration, sometimes the client simply needs the counsellor to let them know that they have heard and have an appreciation of what they have said.

'No.' Ania did not often feel low like this, though it did arise at times, and had done a lot these last few days, since she had recovered those awful memories. Somehow it just didn't seem right, and whilst she tried to feel positive – she had consciously used Maria to try and gain a sense of purpose in her life, it did not sustain her mood. Yes, in her head she knew that Maria gave her a purpose, a reason to be alive, and yet . . .

Debbie sat, aware of the heaviness of the atmosphere in the room, and her sense of Debbie's weightedness as she sat opposite her. She pondered making a further comment, acknowledging once more the difficulty in accepting that she was alive, but thought the better of it. Ania was not repeating it. She clearly was not, at this time, wanting to communicate this again, so it was perhaps best for Debbie to remain present and attentive, holding her feeling of warmth and unconditional positive regard towards Ania, and wait with her in the silence. Debbie knew that whilst outwardly there was silence, inwardly that was probably far from the reality. Silence, she thought, was rarely an empty space.

Ania continued to sit, her thoughts ranging across different images from her past. So many losses, so much grief, so much would never be the same again. Lives shattered, relationships, families, communities. And yet people carried on, found ways to get on with their lives. She knew from the contact she had had with relatives how people were reconstructing their lives. But just at this moment that suddenly seemed like a very distant possibility. Yes, she wanted to go back, she needed to go back, but to what? And wherever she went she would carry her memories with her. She bowed her head and felt an intense sadness and loneliness overwhelm her.

'It is tough for you at the moment, Ania, really hard.'

Ania heard Debbie speaking. Yes, Debbie at least sensed what she was experiencing, though it didn't make it any easier. But she felt an urge to respond, to say something.

'Yes. I wonder if it is all worth it. The struggle. Going home. It feels so big, so much to deal with. I'm tired, Debbie.' She looked up as she spoke, 'I am so tired.'

With that Ania closed her eyes and the tears began to flow. She tightened her eyes, her breath coming in short bursts, her shoulders lifting and dropping as the emotion flowed out of her. She raised her hand to her eyes and rubbed them. Her eyes burned and her throat felt blocked. She felt weak, her arms were numb, her body heavy. She just felt so tired, tired of it all, tired of carrying on, tired of the hurt, of the grief, of the loneliness, of trying to be a good mother when she felt so horrible inside, tired of coming to counselling, tired of . . . , tired of everything. 'It might be better if I was dead.'

Debbie heard the words and stayed with her. 'So much struggle, so tired, leaves you wondering if it would be better if you were dead.'

Clients do feel like dying, do sometimes think it would be better if they were dead. The person-centred counsellor needs to be able to stay with that feeling. It is real and it is valid. People get to what feels like the end of the line, but it does not mean they are about to do harm to themselves. In the moment of disclosure the person-centred counsellor stays with the feelings, empathises with what is present and being experienced by the client. Let the part of the client that wants to die be heard and warmly accepted. Feeling it would be better if you were dead can be a reasonable response to an experience or set of experiences, it is present because of the degree of stress the client is under. We all want to get away from things. Let the client know that you are hearing what they are saying. Often the client needs the depth of their despair to be acknowledged, and through that acknowledgement and warm acceptance of them as a person they may begin to self-question what they have said. But not always. It may be more fixed. The counsellor may want to check whether the client feels safe with themselves, whether there is anything they need from the counsellor.

And of course Ania knew that she didn't really want to be dead, not really, but at the same time the idea of nothing, of just getting away from it all . . . She heard Debbie's response. It was so honest and direct, exactly what she had been thinking and feeling. And yet, yes, she felt that way, but she knew she would struggle on. The truth was, she didn't know any different. You survived. She had to survive. She had a story to tell, a history not to be forgotten, but she was so tired with it all, so tired.

The tears eased and Ania reached over for a tissue, and leaned back into the chair. 'Ohhh.' She let the air blow out of her mouth. 'It's so hard, so hard.'

Debbie nodded and tightened her lips. 'So very hard at the moment.'

'I miss my parents, Debbie, I miss them so much. They were so kind, so loving. They would look after me, but now, I have no one.' She closed her eyes as a wave of grief hit her. 'When I was ill my mother would make soups to warm me up and give me strength. She was always making soups! And she would get me up and make me strong again.' She closed her eyes again as she thought of her brother, how he had been as a teenager, always in trouble. She felt herself smile and then the images of his death swept in and she felt bad about smiling. The tears welled up again. 'Why? Why did it happen, Debbie? Why us? Why me? Why?'

Debbie felt the lump in her own throat and her eyes were watering too. 'I do not know, Ania, I do not know.' She replied in this way because it had been a direct question to her, not just a "Why?" to which she would have empathised.

'They were good people, Debbie, so many good people. It's not right that these things can happen. And no one tried to stop it. The world watched and did nothing, Debbie.'

Debbie felt herself wince. Yes, she was part of that world, what had she done? What could she have done? You live in a so-called free democracy, but what can you do when your government and the international community watch and do so little?

'Yes, you were left to suffer, and only afterwards it seems have we tried to help.'

'And I am grateful, places like this are so good, so important. But . . .'

'Yes, but . . .'

'I would have had my own home and probably been married, and be having children, and spending time with my parents and Tomas, and he'd probably be married too, though he always said that wasn't for him.' She smiled. 'All gone.' She paused. 'All gone.'

Debbie thought of Maria but said nothing. To mention her now would be to direct Ania way from the feelings and the focus that were present for her. As a person-centred counsellor, Debbie trusted Ania's process and stream of thinking and feeling.

'So many possibilities, taken away.'

'I do not know what it will be like when I go back, Debbie, but I know I have to. It will make me sad I am sure, and I must accept that. Perhaps that is my life, to be sad.'

'That how it feels, your life is to be sad?'

'A bit. It is hard to imagine not to feel sad, particularly in a place where there were dreams.'

'Sadness because of the dreams that will not happen.'

Ania nodded. 'They have taken my body, my parents, my brother, and they have taken my dreams.'

'Yes, so much has been taken, and your dreams are a big part of that.'

'I will have to make new dreams, but they will not be the same, they can never be the same.' Ania's eyes watered again, feeling the acute loss of her dreams, her hopes. She did not know why she was feeling it so painfully now, she had known this for a while, but somehow it all seemed so huge all of a sudden.

'No, they will have to be different dreams, not the same ones.'

Ania took a very deep breath, and immediately yawned. 'Oh Debbie, what will become of me, become of us?'

'I wish I knew, Ania, but I know that I hope you have a good life together in your own land, with your own people, speaking your own language.' Her eyes watered again, as she felt the emotion behind the words that she was saying. 'You have touched me so deeply, Ania, and I hear your feelings of tiredness, or feeling you cannot go on with the struggle to live. And I see the proud, courageous, Croatian woman and mother. I wish you well, whatever choices you make, Ania.'

> The reaction from Ania that follows shows that this statement by Debbie is appropriate and timely. There is now no denial of courage. Debbie has summed up many things and Ania has heard them, has found a place in herself from which she can hear what Debbie is saying about her.

Ania had tears in her own eyes, they were different tears. They were different emotions. Her stomach felt knotted as she listened to Debbie and watched the tears welling up in her eyes as she spoke.

'You make me cry again,' Ania smiled and closed her eyes, causing tears to tumble over her eyelids and down her cheeks.

'I make me cry too!' Debbie felt her own tears on one of her cheeks.

The two women sat together for a short while, no words passed between them, and then Ania got up and said she needed a hug. Debbie responded. They held each other, it was a powerful moment for them both. Ania released her grip and stepped back. 'Thank you. I am sorry I felt so weak earlier.'

'That's how you felt, Ania, you have a right to feel that way given all that has happened.'

'Yes, you are right, but I am a mother and I have responsibilities. I should not feel that way. I have a future. Maria is my future. It is her that I must think of.'

'Mhmm, and I want to say "look after yourself too", Ania.'

'Yes, I will.'

Ania lapsed into silence and Debbie waited to hear what she wanted to say next.

'We did not go to the family group last week. I asked Gina to let them know. I was not feeling well enough, but this week we will go.'

'That group has become important for you, for both of you.'

'Yes, it has, and it has helped me to realise that I must go home.'

Debbie nodded, knowing that Ania had made up her mind and was clear about what she needed to do. She admired her for that.

'I admire you for that, Ania.'

'For me it is necessary.'

'Yes. I think I am beginning to understand that more and more as I hear you speak.'

'It is perhaps my English is not good enough?'

'No, no, I didn't mean that, no, it is that I think I can understand a little more the depth of the pull to go home.'

'Yes, I must. It is the right thing to do. And maybe one day I will return to England, when Maria is older. I will make sure she can speak English as well as Croatian. I think that will be very important for her.'

'Yes, I am sure that it will open up possibilities for her.' Debbie paused and glanced at the clock. 'So, we have a while to go today, you want to talk more?'

Ania shook her head. 'I feel like I have said enough today. I have been sad and tearful. And I must make new dreams. I think I would like to go early and surprise Maria. She will not be expecting me, and she will be so pleased.'

Debbie's eyes watered again as she heard Ania's words. Yes, she could imagine the smile on little Maria's face. Somehow, the image really touched her. She did not want Ania to leave with an image of her counsellor all emotional, she wanted her to leave with her sense of wanting to surprise Maria, of looking forward to her reaction, and of anticipating a good experience.

Points for discussion

- What are the main thoughts and feelings that the last counselling session has left you with?

- Where might you have responded differently to Debbie in counselling session 13, and why?
- How would you summarise the quality of Debbie's empathy across the sessions?
- What do you feel are Debbie's strengths as a counsellor, and what are the areas that you feel she might need to develop further?
- What were the key moments in the therapeutic encounters between Ania and Debbie? What made them so significant? What did Debbie contribute to facilitating them?
- If you were to write a report on the therapeutic work done so far with Ania, what would you write?
- What would you be wanting to take to supervision if you were Debbie from the last few counselling sessions?
- Write notes for this session.

Reflections on the process

Debbie's reflections – 'I am filled with emotion after that last session. When Ania said about wanting to go and surprise Maria there was something in the moment that really touched me, and touched me so deeply. It was like, in the midst of all the pain and struggle, loss and doubt, there was hope as well, something to reach out towards, a growth point, if you like. There was something very touching and beautiful in that moment, made more poignant I think because I had met Maria.

'These have been challenging sessions, in the sense that they have made a deep impression on me and drawn my own thoughts and feelings into my awareness. I could not be an effective person-centred counsellor if I was not in touch with, and accurately aware of, my own experiencing. And I am sure there are things that I have missed. I am not a perfect counsellor. I don't think that is possible. I thought I had to be at first, but experience has taught me that I do my best, my best to ensure the core conditions are offered to every client.

'So many emotions, so many feelings, so much to come to terms with, so much horror. I see it every day that I work at the centre, of course, so many people are affected by war. The numbers are astonishing and to think globally for a moment, the number of people affected by the horror of war must be vast. So much pain.

'I cannot change the big picture and I accept that, although I did wince when Ania talked of how the world had sat and watched the war in Bosnia. I hope we have learned and it will not be that way again, but it continues in too many other parts of the world. I do what I can with the people and the families that I see. When people have been the victims of inhumanity – and I want to say that whilst some are victims, others I would describe more as targets, having been singled out for particular acts of atrocity and inhumanity –

I strongly believe that what they need is to be exposed to a sense of humanity. That is what I offer – myself. That is all I am and all that I have.

'From my own experience, I am sure that it helps my female clients that I am a woman. There is a sense of female solidarity that often emerges, that whilst I have not experienced what my clients describe, because I am a woman my presence has greater significance. For Ania I think that it was also my presence as a mother although that was not outwardly discussed. I still feel sure that it somehow set a particular tone to my responding when issues related to Maria were being addressed or referred to.

'Key moments in the sessions? Strange, really, nothing stands out and yet there is also a sense that everything stands out. The physical contact was important. I don't think I am skilled enough in body work to apply that to my clients whose bodies, as well as their emotions, have been traumatised by warfare. I do wonder whether this is an area I need to develop. The thought of offering bodily empathy to bodily trauma is an area I know little about, yet I know colleagues who have looked into this. It is not only hearts and minds that must grieve, and release their anguish and pain, so too must the actual physical self.

'And hearing Ania talk in her own language, yes, that was important. She was able to be more expressive and I think that was important. I am glad that I invited her to say it in her own words, although I can't remember whether I did, or whether she just started speaking in Croatian. We think in our own language and we attach meaning to our feelings in the words of our own language. Perhaps to release those feelings we need the language by which we know them.

'Ania has changed over the weeks and months. She has blossomed, although things became very difficult just recently with the recovered memories. I had begun to sense something, but was not clear as to what it would be. It is so important not to introduce anything to encourage these memories to the surface. The client has to trust the counsellor, but more importantly, perhaps, their own internal system or process must have reached a point at which the experiences need to come into awareness. Perhaps it is governed by when the structure of self can no longer keep them hidden, that there is a some kind of inward pressure – maybe the actualising tendency – forcing them to awareness in order to establish greater wholeness in a self-structure that has become split or fragmented. Or maybe there is something that becomes recognised within the person that they can now hold the experience that has been concealed. And maybe it is some of both.

'I know Ania will return to Croatia and maybe to Bosnia, and I know it will not be easy for her, or for Maria. It will bring up so much for Ania I am sure, but she will perhaps be in the best place to take her own healing process forward. Is it for the best? I do not know. Who can say? What is important, as I felt in the sessions as this became more and more of a topic and a possibility, is that Ania makes a decision based on what she believes to be best, and so long as it is emerging from her own congruent experiencing and her own internal locus of evaluation. I trust her to know what she needs to do, and I do not say that lightly.

'How much longer we will work together, I do not know. Perhaps it will depend on when Ania leaves? Maybe we will work together until that time, and my role will then be to listen to her as she works through issues related to endings and beginnings.

'So, whilst I remain horrified by what people can do to others, and in particular the horrors men inflict on women, though not exclusively so, I am inspired by the courage and the determination of people like Ania to "do what is necessary" to live on in spite of their experiences.'

Ania's reflections – 'It was not easy to talk at first. You get out of the habit of talking about difficult things. I have a lot of pain, a lot of bad memories. I accept that I will always have them. But it makes me to not want to forget. For me, the counselling has been important, but not easy. I cannot always express what I feel. It was good to talk in my own language. That was important to me. And maybe I will need to do that again. I speak my own language at the family group. It feels good for me to do this.

'Feelings have their own language and you do not always need to say the words. I can see in Debbie's eyes that she is feeling so much. I do not want to hurt her, but I have to make my feelings known to her. I have to come and release them. For too long I, as you say, bottled them up. Debbie said it was like bursting a boil and it is so. Yes, and I think I have not yet got out all of the poison. One day I hope that I will. But I will not forget.

'I have to go home. It pulls, and the pull grows. I do not know how it will be. But I did not know how it would be when I came to England, and I was feeling worse then. I had just lost so much. Now I can maybe make a new start, with Maria, and maybe I can help people in my own country. I can understand why counselling is important. But I think it would be better for people to talk to people from their own country, and in their own language. Perhaps one day I can do that? I would be very pleased to do that.

'I have good days and bad, that is how it is. But I have a few more friends now with the family group and Maria is growing up all the time. I want to be back in Croatia before she begins school. I want her to have time to adjust.

'I want to thank Debbie. How she has been has made a difference. Having someone to listen, really listen, someone who does not judge me – these are important to me. I do not know how she learned to be that way, but I am glad that she is. And it is how I would like to be as well.

'But now I must make preparations and arrangements. It will be a busy time, but I will continue to see Debbie. That is important to me.'

Maria's reflections – 'I like Debbie. She helps mama. Sometimes mama is sad. She cries sometimes. But she is happy when she is with me. So I like to be with mama to make her happy.'

PART 2

Graham confronts his memories

He'd never forget the smell. The scene was bad enough; the bodies, bloodied and mutilated, piled up and rotting, but it was the smell that haunted him . . .

CHAPTER 10

Counselling session 1: accepting the need to talk

Graham was sitting in the waiting room, it was a Tuesday afternoon and quite quiet in the village surgery. He was thumbing through a magazine, wondering in his own mind what he was doing there. He had been reluctant to come, it wasn't something he really saw himself as needing. He was 40 years of age, 20 years in the army, the only life he had known, really. He had come out of the army two years ago and at first all had seemed OK. He'd got a job in security. It hadn't been easy to settle into civilian life, but he had held the job down, but the last six months had become something of a nightmare. He'd lost his confidence, felt low, suffered anxiety attacks, couldn't sleep and now he was on sick leave, and had been referred to see a counsellor at his GP surgery.

His GP, Dr Cross, had been very good. He had said that he thought he had things he needed to talk over, perhaps from the past. Graham regarded himself as a good judge of men, and trusted his first impressions. Dr Cross seemed to be someone who was quite clear and matter of fact – he liked that. Didn't have time for woolliness and uncertainty. He was used to clarity.

He'd never been to counselling before, seemed to him something that people went to who were weak-minded in some way, people who couldn't cope, who needed a shoulder to cry on. He didn't cry. You didn't cry. He'd seen buddies die, he'd seen them buried. No one cried. It was selfish. You showed respect. You kept your feelings to yourself. You didn't cry. But he had to admit that he felt a need to talk things over with someone, but was clear that it would be 'man-to-man', he just wanted some direction, what to do, and then he'd get on with his life again. Maybe he should go home, sort himself out. Maybe this wasn't the place for him. He was about to put the magazine down and head home when he heard his name.

'Mr Barlow?' He heard his name and looked up.

'Yes, that's me.' He closed the magazine and placed it back on the table as he stood up.

'Hello, my name's Oliver. We spoke briefly last week to arrange the appointment. Good to meet you.' Oliver extended his hand. Graham took it and gripped him.

Oliver noted the strength of the grip and the sweatiness of Graham's palm. Maybe a bit anxious, he thought to himself, though it was a warm day, but certainly a very matter-of-fact kind of handshake. Oliver lessened his grip and their hands parted.

'Would you like to follow me, the counselling room is just along the corridor.'

'Certainly, thank you.' Graham followed Oliver and walked through the door that Oliver had opened for him. He put aside his thought of going home, at least for the moment. As he looked around the room he noticed that it was not very large, there was a couple of comfortable looking green chairs, and a couple of Monet prints on the walls, a small table with a table lamp, and a window at the far end.

'Where shall I sit?'

'Whichever. Up to you.'

Graham was slightly surprised, he was used to people having their own seats and, well, being directed to where he should sit.

'Oh, right, um, OK, I'll sit here.'

'Sure, please, sit down.'

Graham sat in the chair in the corner with the window on his right, and opposite the door. He didn't think about it, but in fact it was a choice conditioned by his training and his army experiences. He always sat facing the door, when he had a choice, avoiding having his back to an entrance. That was how it was. It was so much a part of him that he didn't give it a moment's thought.

'So, let me begin by saying a little about counselling, what it is and what you might expect from it, and if you have any questions then please, ask away.'

'OK.' Graham had no idea what to expect, but he felt at ease with having time to listen to what Oliver had to tell him.

Oliver talked about what counselling was, and described the nature and the limits of confidentiality.

That all seemed clear to Graham, particularly when he mentioned about the need to break confidentiality if, for instance, someone was disclosing intent to harm others as, for instance as a result of an act of terrorism.

'Yes, I should bloody well hope so', was Graham's response.

'Obviously something you feel passionate about?'

Graham nodded, '20 years in the military, I've seen a few things, things I'd rather forget, but I know the damage those kinds of bombs can do to people. I know what it can be like.' Graham's jaw was set firm as he finished speaking, and as he consciously pushed aside images in his head. Everyone had memories and you had to learn to deal with them.

'Mhmm, having not had that experience myself I can only imagine what it must be like, but you do, you've seen the effects first hand and *know* what it's like.'

'Northern Ireland, Bosnia, the Gulf War, yes, I've been there, seen scenes that, well, you wouldn't choose to see, but comes with the job. You get on with it.'

Oliver nodded. 'Mhmm, yeah, you get on with it.'

Graham felt quite OK as he spoke. Felt as though he was talking about things that he knew about – on his own territory, so to speak.

'Most do. Some can't and they don't usually carry on.'

'But you found your own way to get on with it.'

'Well, you're part of a group, you're there for each other. It's a tough life, but it gives you a lot. Toughens you up. Makes you independent, but it also makes you a part of a team, aware of the need to trust, to act when ordered and be ready to support your comrades.'

'Mhmm, quite an experience, toughening, independent and being part of a team like that.'

'You place your life in their hands, you have to trust them, and they have to trust you. There can't be any weakness, any hesitancy, everyone has to know what they are doing, and get on with it. Companies are as strong as the weakest link, and in life and death situations you don't want a weak link.'

Graham wondered just how much Oliver really did understand about what he was saying. He'd already indicated that he could only imagine what it was like. Could he? Could anyone? Too many fucking awful films. No, he thought, as he looked over at Oliver, you haven't got the first fucking clue what I'm talking about.

Graham is basing his thoughts on what Oliver has said. Was Oliver right to have talked of not having had Graham's experience? He was being open and honest. But he has to earn Graham's respect if the relationship is to become therapeutically productive. Graham will need to feel that Oliver can relate to him man-to-man. A client's respect for their counsellor might be considered a requirement for effective therapeutic process.

Oliver was aware that the counselling session was still very much in its early phase, and he was already getting quite a sense of Graham as a person. He was very aware of the quite matter-of-fact style that Graham expressed himself through. He sought to mirror that himself.

'Mhmm. Weak links are bad news for everyone.'

Graham nodded, and lapsed into silence. He wasn't sure what to say next, and Oliver didn't seem to be saying anything more. It felt strange, not like a normal conversation. He wasn't sure what to make of it. He needed some answers, and his way of dealing with a situation like that would be to ask questions.

The therapeutic relationship has begun with the counsellor demonstrating empathy for the client's thoughts and ideas. It is very matter of fact. The counsellor stays with this, not trying to push the client towards feelings, but accepting him as he is, as he chooses to be. But now it has reached a point at which the client has to find his own direction. He responds by asking questions.

'So, what happens then, what happens now? What do we talk about?'

'Well, that's up to you. The way I work is to really offer a space here for people to talk about whatever is important for them. I don't know what you need to talk about, or bring into the counselling. That's up to you. My role is to communicate my understanding of what you are telling me, what you are experiencing, being open to my reactions, being up front with you about what I might experience. I don't see myself as an expert on your life, or anyone else's.'

Graham listened. 'Sounds a bit vague to me. So you just listen, and I have to decide what to talk about?'

'That's pretty much how it is.'

'I don't know what to talk about. I was hoping you'd give me some answers.'

'OK, that's a good place to start, you saw the doctor, he suggested you come and talk to me, and for you what you wanted and expected was to get a few answers, yes?'

'Yes.'

Silence again. Oliver considered the situation. He could let the silence remain, but would that really be communicating empathy to what Graham was clearly saying that he wanted? Would it be therapeutically helpful to stay with the silence? It didn't feel like a very therapeutic silence, more awkward with an overlay of irritation in the air.

'And it would be bloody irritating, to say the least, if you found you didn't get those answers?'

'Well yes.'

> Perhaps a slight hesitancy from the client, maybe slightly taken aback by the counsellor's forthright response. The silence has been broken as it did not feel to the counsellor that it was therapeutically valuable. He is seeking to be empathic to the client, to the voiced need for answers.

'OK, so you want answers. And I guess that means you have some questions.'

'I want to know what I need to do to get myself back to work, back to feeling myself again.'

'Mhmm, it's being unable to get to work and not feeling yourself, and what to do about it, that's really on your agenda?'

Graham nodded.

'And this is something new for you to deal with, do you mind if I call you Graham?'

'No, that's fine.'

'OK, so this is a new experience for you, Graham?'

'Yes, I mean, what have I got to be concerned about? I have a lovely home, my wife, three children, the job is fine, nothing there is a problem, but I sit at home and just feel like I don't want to face anything. Everything's an effort. I feel tired all of the time, can't seem to motivate myself. I potter around the house, but not really getting much done. Can't get into a routine. Had one, but not now. It's frustrating the hell out of Angela, my wife. I just can't seem to get hold of myself, and, well, it was Angela who persuaded me to see the doctor a few weeks back, and he said maybe I needed some time out, maybe it was stress, though what I have to be stressed about . . .' His voice trailed off as he shook his head. He looked, and felt, pissed off with the whole thing.

'So, everything is an effort and really you just feel like you can't motivate yourself to get anything done, you say that you can't seem to get a hold of yourself?'

'Like I can't . . .' Graham clenched his fists, raising his arms slightly as he sat in the chair. 'Just can't get a grip, somehow.'

'Mhmm, yeah, can't get a grip.' Oliver reflected back the physical movement as he spoke, and something of the facial expression as well.

'I deal with things, that's me, that's my nature. There's a problem and I find the solution and sort it. Job done. Move on to the next thing . . .'

'Mhmm.'

'. . . but I'm not doing that.' Graham could feel the frustration building up inside himself. And he was tired as well, it was like he was frustrated and too tired to feel frustrated both at the same time.

'Not being able to find a solution, and so you can't move on to the next thing.'

'I faff about, just can't seem to settle on anything.'

'Mhmm, so there's a difficulty in settling on any one thing.' Oliver nodded as he spoke, maintaining the eye contact that had developed in recent minutes.

Graham shook his head and tightened his jaw. 'I just, oh I don't know, doctor said he might put me on some pills, but I said no, don't believe in it.'

'So you're not taking anything at the moment?'

'No, and I don't want to.'

'Pills aren't something you want to take, at least, not for something like this?'

'Why can't I . . . , oh I don't know, I just want to get back to how I was. And I think talking about it will make fuck all difference.'

'Frustrating the fuck out of you. How you were, being able to get on with things.'

'Deal with things, you know, get things done.'

'Yeah, get things done. That's really important to you, Graham, I can see that.' Oliver did not stray away from empathising with what Graham was saying. He knew there were causes to what was happening for Graham, but at the moment Graham was focusing on his frustration and his desire to get back to being how he was. He would trust that other material would emerge when it was right for Graham to express it.

Oliver is matching Graham's language, staying with him, mirroring his style of talking directly to the point. Style of empathy is an important consideration, it is not merely the words that are spoken or the facial expression as the empathic response is communicated. Oliver is keeping pace with Graham in a number of ways, allowing him the opportunity to settle into the exchange. It will all help to establish the language and style of communication. It tells the client to say it as he wants to say it, that the counsellor isn't going to use language, or avoid language, that might cause the client to feel uneasy about how they want to express themselves.

'So, why am I like this? And why now?'

'Mhmm, why like you are, and why now?'

'I don't know. I'm not sleeping well. I wake up and I'm tired. Some days I really struggle to get up. I don't feel interested in anything. I feel like there's an empty space in my head sometimes.'

'Mhmm, like an empty space . . .' Oliver frowned. 'That how it feels now?'

'Not so much. No. Funny, it actually feels quite good to talk even though it feels like I haven't said anything.' Graham tightened his lips.

'So, talking like this seems to leave you feeling quite good?'

'Hmm, I don't know why, haven't got any answers.'

'No, well, no answers, but something good about talking like this.' Oliver was aware of wondering whether Graham had talked much at all about what he was feeling and experiencing. He recognised it as his own curiosity and put aside any notion of asking the question of Graham, choosing instead to allow the silence that had developed to remain, leaving Graham, with whatever thoughts and feelings that were present for him following their exchange about his feeling good.

Graham felt a pressure to talk. He wasn't sure what he wanted to say, but he felt a need to say something. 'It's not been easy, adjusting to civilian life.'

'No.' Oliver thought about reflecting back what Graham had said but felt it was perhaps unnecessary.

This is an interesting situation. Communicating empathy is not about exhaustively repeating back what a client says. In this case it is to be taken that the client has a sense that what he has said has been heard. The counsellor recognises this. Sometimes, as in this case, a kind of empathic summary can be used to confirm what has been heard.

'Particularly after 20 years.'

Oliver wondered if there was any training available within the military to help people deal with the transition, but he put the thought aside.

'Twenty years is a long time, and a lot to adjust to.'

'Yes, it is.' Graham pushed aside images from those years. Yes, there had been good times, great times, but those were not the images that came to mind. He didn't want to start talking about them now. He'd rather not think about them. But he felt suddenly hot, sweaty, and his heart was pounding. It did that a lot these days, often for no apparent reason. He could be out somewhere and would come over in a sweat, even feel light-headed. He put it down to his age. Doctor had told him his blood pressure was up – not to the point that he needed medication, but he needed to watch it, take more exercise, watch his diet.

'You look deep in thought, 20 years of memories?'

'Hmm? Oh, yes, something like that.'

Oliver sensed that somehow the silence now was more natural, easier. Not comfortable, but it felt somehow as though it was more timely and not borne out of awkwardness.

Graham was looking towards the door. It wasn't that he was thinking of leaving, the reality was that he wasn't thinking at all. He was aware of sitting, but his eyes felt so heavy. He sat up and stretched, taking a deep breath as he did so. Again, tight-lipped.

'It just feels from here that there's a lot going on for you at the moment on the inside, and it leaves you finding it hard to focus on the outside.' Oliver spoke from a strong sense of Graham spending a lot of time with thoughts and feelings. It wasn't something he had planned to say, but it felt very present for him as he sat observing Graham.

Oliver has spoken from his own experience of the relationship with Graham. It has not come out of a pressure to speak, or to get out of an awkward silence. It is a view that has arisen in his mind that seemed, to Oliver, to sum up what he was picking up from Graham. Is it an intervention consistent with person-centred practice? Oliver is working at the therapeutic relationship, with connection, with conveying to Graham his appreciation of what he is saying and experiencing.

Graham thought about what Oliver had just said. A lot going on in the inside, that was true. He did spend a lot of time thinking about things, and it probably contributed to him not getting a firm hold on himself. He hadn't planned to say anything specifically, the words just came out. 'Memories, you know?'

'Memories can be intrusive.'

It seemed to Graham that perhaps Oliver might be a man that he could relate to. At least he seemed to say what he thought, he made sense. He liked that. Yes, he felt a little more at ease in one sense, though he also felt uneasy as well, but that was more linked to the memories in his head and the idea that he was sitting here with a counsellor.

'I've seen too much, Oliver, been to too many places, seen too much of the inhumanity that people inflict on one another. It's a brutal world out there, a brutal world.'

'Mhmm, yeah, too many things, the brutal side of the world.'

'Far too much.' Graham didn't want to describe what he had seen. He knew it was shocking, he didn't need to fill Oliver's head with it. No, they were military memories and he needed to keep them to the military world, his world, his inner world, or with old colleagues, but not outside of the military. You didn't speak about things outside of the regiment, that had been ingrained in him over the years, and it remained a dominant factor.

They lapsed back into silence. For Graham it felt as though he had gone as far as he could. For Oliver there was a profound sense that Graham had more to say but for the present seemed unable to say it. He respected that. You know what you know, Oliver thought to himself as he sat opposite Graham, and why should you tell me after, well, 40 minutes of a counselling session?

Graham suddenly looked across at Oliver. 'They aren't the kind of things you talk about.' Graham spoke in a very direct and matter-of-fact tone of voice. It was somehow quite stark and intrusive to the silence that had developed.

Oliver heard the words and yet felt that somehow, somewhere, there was a tone in Graham's voice that sounded as though maybe he was asking permission to talk about them, or was it his fantasy? He could imagine that perhaps part of Graham might want to talk, and maybe that part was kept under wraps. 'No, not the kind of things you usually talk about.'

It may seem a small thing but the inclusion of the word 'usually' is indicative of an empathic response that goes beyond the words Graham has used. It recognises that Graham does not usually talk about the things that he is thinking. It conveys an invitation to say more, because whilst it is not something to talk about usually, counselling is not a place for the usual kind of conversation.

'You'd have to be there to understand.'

'My not being there, or in some similar situation, you mean?'

Graham nodded. 'Not easy, and I'm not sure that it would do any good to talk about them.'

'That somehow talking about them won't make any difference?'

'Probably make it worse.'

'Mhmm, talking about your memories would make it worse, or maybe make you feel worse.'

'I'd feel worse. Can't change the memories, they'll be the same.'

'So, sharing those memories won't change them, and could make you feel worse.'

Graham tightened his jaw.

Oliver had noticed the time a couple of minutes previously, and knew they had less than ten minutes left. He wasn't going to mention the time, not just yet, it would, or at least could, divert Graham's attention from the focus that had developed for him, a focus that Oliver fully trusted as having emerged for a reason. He didn't want to mention the time and possibly direct Graham into a place where he pulled back and prepared to end, not just yet anyway.

'It's tiring to think about it, it really is. It did feel better a short while ago, but now, well, now it doesn't. I'm not sure what I am getting out of this.'

'Tiredness after feeling better a short while ago.'

'I just want an answer, I want someone to tell me what to do.'

'Mhmm. That's how it is. You want someone to tell you what to do.' Oliver paused. 'It's what you are used to, I imagine.'

'You're not going to tell me, are you?'

'No, not because I know and am keeping something back, but because first I don't give advice, and second, if I did it's hard to tell someone what to do when you don't know the full story.'

'Yeah, I can see that. But you must see lots of people like me?'

'No, I see lots of people, but everyone's different, everyone has their own questions, and their own answers.'

'No fancy psychological remedy then?'

'No.'

Graham sort of appreciated the frankness, though it still frustrated him. 'So it's up to me, isn't it?'

Oliver nodded, feeling suddenly as though there had been a shift, a movement.

'I need answers but I don't know where to find them. And I'm not sure I have the energy to start looking.'

'That's really clear, have you the energy to look for the answers.'

Graham shook his head, his lips were tight once again. Oliver was so aware of the tension that Graham must be carrying, so much effort going in to maintaining that facial expression. 'I need to do something. I can't go without doing something, getting something.'

'Mhmm, you know you need to do something. What do you want to do, Graham?' Oliver spoke quite softly, not directly empathising with what had been said, but rather acknowledging Graham's realisation by focusing on the implication. He felt warm acceptance of Graham, a man not used to talking but now desperately needing to but unable to. Yes, Oliver felt his unconditional positive regard for Graham was genuinely heartfelt.

It is vital that unconditional positive regard is not so much an attitude of mind but more a quality of heart within the therapeutic relationship. When this is the case it is a very powerful factor in encouraging psychological change in the client. The role of the heart in effective therapy is an area that needs greater exploration. The person-centred approach captures it to some degree by having unconditional positive regard as a core condition. But perhaps there are hidden depths to what this means that remain to be more fully explored and understood.

Graham felt strangely still for a moment. He took a deep breath and heard himself speaking. 'I need to talk, don't I?'

Oliver nodded, short, quick nods.

'I need to talk about things.'

Oliver nodded again. 'When you're ready, and at your own pace, and in your own way.'

Graham smiled slightly as he shook his head again. 'That's what today has been about, hasn't it, me realising I have to talk.'

'That how it seems?'

'Yes, but there isn't time now.' He took a deep breath. 'Have to wait a week now.'

'Yes, we only have a few minutes, and I don't want to encourage or discourage you from saying anything. The time's yours, I just want to check out that you want to continue coming?'

'Yes, I don't understand this, but yes, I do. I feel like you're someone I can maybe talk to, I don't know, at least, I felt that earlier, now I feel different, I can't describe it, different.' He went tight-lipped again.

The session drew to a close with both men agreeing on the time for the next appointment and dates for succeeding appointments at least for the next five weeks.

Graham left the counselling session feeling a little woolly himself, and still quite tired. He felt he needed time to sit on his own. He took himself off for a short walk and sat on a bench overlooking the fields. He closed his eyes and lost all track of time. Half an hour had passed by the time he got up and headed back to get his car and drive home.

Oliver sat in the counselling room writing his notes and being with what he was experiencing in response to his time with Graham. He was quite pleased with the session. He recognised that people could not be expected to 'tell-all' during a first session. Why should they, unless it was so pressing that the person could no longer contain it. And he had experienced sessions like that, sometimes the person never coming back for a second session, as though they had unloaded, taken the pressure off, and then tried to get on with their lives again.

Graham wasn't going to be like that. It felt to Oliver that Graham really had realised that he needed to talk and he, Oliver, was left to imagine what Graham had witnessed – possibly even perpetrated – in a military career that now seemed to have come back to haunt him, assuming it had ever left him.

Points for discussion

- Evaluate the effectiveness of Oliver's use of self in the session. There were times when he voiced the content of his own awareness, and times when he didn't. Why was this?
- From the perspective of person-centred theory, when is it likely to be most therapeutically helpful for a counsellor to communicate what they are thinking or feeling?
- Trace Graham's changing views on the idea of needing counselling through the session. Have they changed and, if so, what factors have enabled this change to occur?
- What are your fantasies about Graham's past? How will you ensure they will not distort your hearing of what Graham has to say when he begins to share his past?
- What enabled Graham to realise that he needed to talk about his past?

- Evaluate Oliver's application of the person-centred approach in this opening session.
- Do you have prejudices against military personnel? If a counsellor did, what should they do about it?
- Write notes for this session.

CHAPTER 11

Counselling session 2: memories of a violent and personal death

Graham was sitting down, aware that the past week had, if anything, been more
difficult. And it seemed to him that the last counselling session had contributed
to that. But he knew that he needed to talk though he wasn't going to talk
about all of it. He was trained, he was a professional, he had been taught to
deal with these things and not to say anything. Yet here he was, contemplating
sharing memories, images, that had been so much an accepted part of his life,
part of himself, and which now had come to feel more like unwelcome intrusions into his thoughts and his dreams.

'So, good to see you again. How do you want to use our time today, Graham?'
Oliver had sat himself down and was sitting upright in his chair, looking somewhat expectant and wanting to get on with it, whatever "it" was, Graham
thought to himself.

Graham took a deep breath. 'Hard to know where to begin, but I know I have to.
I guess start at the beginning, at least, where I first started to see things, witness
events that are still very much with me.'

'OK, take your time, Graham, and only tell me what you want to say.'

'Belfast. We all knew we'd spend time there, and we all knew that we were trained
to cope – and we were – but it wasn't easy, always watching your back, always
aware that something could happen at any time, to any one of us. Funny thing is,
I like the Irish people, always have, regardless of which side of the religious
divide. And yet, in the uniform you were immediately the enemy to a great
many people.'

'Sounds like everything changes the moment you put on the uniform in that
context.'

'Yeah, and, you know, that was how it was, you accepted it, you got on with it.
But it wasn't quite how I expected it. I guess it was the first time I saw the
bloody aftermath of terrorism, "the troubles" as the Irish like to describe it.'
Graham shook his head. 'It's strange, really, you go through so much and you
do all that you can to avoid feeling anything. You get a physical reaction,
seeing bodies blown apart can be physically sickening, but the emotion, you

can't afford to let that get to you so you keep away from it. You work hard, you keep your focus, you have to. You all do it. That's how it is.'

'Mhmm, focus and work to cope. The carnage was physically sickening, but the emotions are contained.' Oliver maintained a very to the point tone of voice.

Graham swallowed. 'Yeah. They have to be. You can't have emotions in combat situations.' He paused, shaking his head slightly as he did so. 'And what gets me is the futility of it all. Years and years of bloody confrontation – and it still goes on with the punishment beatings – and people just cannot, will not, let go and learn to accept each other.' Graham shook his head. 'And I'm not surprised. There's no forgiveness. I've seen it elsewhere, people who cannot let go of the past, cannot let go of history, cannot draw a line under, yes, horrifying events, but unless someone starts drawing that line, what happens? It just carries on. And even if the violence eases, people's hearts and minds are full of it, waiting for something to trigger it off again.'

Oliver nodded. He felt similar sentiments, but he wasn't there to discuss these. Graham clearly felt passionate and he wanted to acknowledge it.

The counsellor notes his thoughts and feelings and chooses not to mention them. Rather he responds to the note of passion and caring in Graham's voice.

'It's something you really care deeply about.'

'I've seen the effects, communities tearing themselves apart. People, tearing each other apart. Death, broken bodies. And for what? ' He shook his head again.

'And for what . . .' Oliver spoke softly not wishing to in any way disturb the flow of thoughts, and perhaps feelings, that were present for Graham.

Graham took another deep breath and made to begin to speak, but stopped, looking to his left. He realised he didn't know what to say. He drew another deep breath and sighed.

'Not easy, huh?'

'It's like another world. It destroys your faith in humanity. We were first on the scene at a bombing. Legs, arms, guts, bloodied stains on the walls – what was left of them. The first time, it just didn't feel real, and it was, but you couldn't take it in. And you couldn't stop to try to take it in, you were on duty, there was always the risk of a second bomb.'

Oliver realised that he had no concept of what such a scene would look like or how he would feel witnessing it, yet he had to convey an appreciation of what Graham was telling him. 'Unreal, and yet terribly real, and no time to process it.'

'No, no you can't do things like that. You have to be alert. You have to remember all that you have learned. You're looking out for your buddy, for the team, and they're looking out for you. No time to feel, and I guess you do harden up. You do begin to accept it as "normal". And at the time, at the time then it didn't feel normal, but over the years, well, maybe it began to feel normal, but looking back now, I wonder at myself, at what I became. And yet, it was right, it was the only way to cope.'

'Hardening up and accepting it all as normal, and you wonder at it, and at yourself.'

'It was a mess over there.' Graham looked up and met Oliver's eyes. He was searching, though he wasn't sure for what. Oliver returned his gaze. Graham knew Oliver had not seen what he had seen, but he wasn't flinching in the eye contact. He respected that. 'So much misinformation, you did your duty, tried to keep yourself and your mates safe. But the people, the amount of venom, poison between the two communities.' Graham shook his head and looked away. 'Kids, women, as well as the men. And there were some brave people who did seek to foster goodwill. Some didn't survive.' He returned to the eye contact. 'I had two tours over there.'

Graham stopped, he'd lost a few good mates. 'When you've got someone hurt, badly hurt, and you're trying to get them away, but the petrol bombs are still flying, and the bricks, you wonder – not at the time, you can't afford to – but later, you wonder, what are these people about? And we weren't saints either. But we had a job to do, try and create order, try and bring some kind of security to the place. I've seen people shot who didn't need to have been, and beatings that shouldn't have happened. And, yes, I was part of that as well. It happens.'

Oliver nodded, aware that for the moment Graham was concentrating on telling the story rather than being his feelings about it all. That was OK. Graham, needed to tell it in his own way, feelings could come later. For now, the story needed to be told. And he needed to convey acceptance towards Graham, for who he was. He did accept him. It was strange, as he had said about things that didn't need to happen, he didn't feel any kind of judgement. How could he? Would he have been any different in the same circumstances?

The military person who has experienced combat can only speak in his own way, tell his story in his own words. It will come about in ways that reflect a lack of trust for civilians and a need to hide the deep, emotional impact of war. There will be a need for self-protection in all of this. There will be a feeling, perhaps, of not wanting to talk to someone who does not understand, who cannot have the first clue exactly what it is that is being talked about. This is the challenge to the counsellor of any theoretical persuasion, and a reason why war veterans may prefer to choose a counsellor with military experience.

Above all else, the counsellor *must* be authentic and focused. And there must be warm acceptance of the client being from a military background conveyed to and experienced by them. The person-centred counsellor has to enter the client's inner world and frame of reference, and that is likely to feel very different from what they may have encountered elsewhere.

'Yeah, found yourself wondering what the people were about, and why things happened.'

Graham nodded, 'yeah, things happened. It was war, whatever the politicians said. Civil war, maybe, but still war. So much fucking hatred, and we had a job to do and we did it, my God we did it, and we have to be proud for that, trying to keep the two communities apart. You know, part of me wants to say "in that God-forsaken place", but the irony is it is all rooted in religion.' He shook his head. 'You can't think like this at the time, you can't let your feelings overwhelm you.'

'No, have to keep focused, yeah, keep safe, mind your backs, do the job, get out.' It wasn't empathy for Graham's words, but was an empathy for the spirit of what Oliver felt he was communicating, though it only captured some of it.

You can't always capture everything, and the counsellor judges in a split second what is the most important factors to communicate. Often it is instinctive. Sometimes it is coloured by elements within the counsellor, or particular sensitivities, as certain things said by a client make a stronger impression.

Training, work on increasing self-awareness, supervision should all contribute to the counsellor being able to be accurately responsive to the key comments made by their clients.

Graham was suddenly feeling a lot of emotion. It happened, but he usually kept it to himself. It was Geordie. He felt water in his eyes and told himself not to. For fuck's sake, he said to himself in his head, you're a fucking soldier. And you don't show emotion.

Oliver noticed the expression on Graham's face start to harden, his jaw had tightened noticeably. Yes, something inside him said that what he was seeing now was his military bearing. It was how Graham needed to be, how the military person had to be, and he accepted that. Couldn't get much different, he thought to himself, between the military person holding his emotions under check, and the person-centred counsellor whose emotional sensitivity is what he brings into his relationships with clients. And yet both, in their own way, were disciplined. Mhmm. He made sure his attention was on Graham.

Emotion will not be shown easily. It is not something that a military person is going to reveal, and certainly not to another man unless they really cannot contain it. There are no tears shed in combat, or at the funeral services of comrades in arms. The counsellor must be able to work with this, accept this as a necessary way of being which, whilst it will serve its purpose in a military context, can lead to emotional difficulties later, when the military discipline may no longer be so present to contain what is felt but not expressed. Many war veterans do turn to drugs and alcohol, but that is by no means to suggest that all do. And the suicide rate amongst war veterans is high, over 20 per year among Falkland veterans over the 20 years since the conflict.

Graham was thinking back. He and Geordie had been close mates, they just got on well and spent a lot of time on and off duty together. He took a deep breath and could feel the emotion, and his eyes beginning to water. He didn't want to talk about it. He never had. You didn't. Geordie wouldn't have wanted him to talk about it. Geordie was free now, in heaven somewhere, and probably having a good time, knowing him. He didn't want to talk about it, didn't want to show emotion, and certainly not to another man, even if he was a counsellor.

Oliver, having seen the change in Graham's expression, knew that he was experiencing something, and something that caused him to harden his expression. He decided to respond to what he felt was being communicated to him, at least his understanding of it. He chose to speak in a matter of fact way to empathise with how Graham was likely to be about it.

'Memories. Things you don't want to talk to me about.'

Graham looked Oliver in the eyes. It was a hard and searching look. It was the look of a man who was trying to know if the other could be trusted. For Graham there was already a knowing that Oliver could never be trusted in the same way as members in his company could be. That kind of trust didn't exist outside the military. Putting your life on the line, and having others' lives trusted to you. You were a team, a unit. You trusted, it welded you together. This counsellor could never offer him that. He continued to look at Oliver.

Oliver held the eye contact. He knew instinctively, and from his understanding of military processes, that this was an important and perhaps defining moment. What he said now, how he was experienced by Graham now, would perhaps set the tone for what was to follow. It could have a facilitative effect, or it could put up a barrier. He realised he was nodding, ever so slightly, his own jaw had tightened as well.

There was something about Oliver's expression, the firmness in his facial expression, his steady eye contact, something, he wasn't sure what, but he began to talk. 'There was this one day, we were heading off to a security incident, we were in the second vehicle. Geordie was in the first. Hit a mine ...' Graham paused. The explosion was enormous. He could still hear it. He was still looking at Oliver, steadily, searchingly. 'I held him and he died in my arms, first time I'd experienced that. He was bleeding really badly, nothing anyone could do. Shrapnel had ripped him open. He held me, such a tight grip, hanging on, hanging on to life, looking at me, pleading, but he couldn't speak. I can still feel him holding me, and then his grip lessened and he'd gone. For me, that was the worst, at least, the worst then.' A tear seeped over his eyelid.

'Your best mate, dying in that way, in your arms, feeling him holding on to you
   . . .' Oliver maintained eye contact and facial expression.

> A hard empathic response, holding Graham on his experience of Geordie
> dying in his arms. Oliver maintains his bearing. He is showing empathy
> through his physical bearing. It's an important moment.

Graham nodded. He could see it still. He knew he'd never forget it, however many
   other 'incidents' there had been in his military career, that had been his first
   close up and personal experience of death.
'Memories and feelings.'
Graham was swallowing hard, the emotion burned in his throat, his stomach was
   tight, he closed his eyes which pushed out more teardrops. 'You don't cry, you
   absorb it, use it in a controlled way in the next battle.'
'That how it was for you?'
Graham nodded. 'It built up in us all, that's why things happen. You bottle it up
   and, well, sometimes you can let it go, but sometimes it stays, builds up and,
   bang, something happens, someone shoots when they had no business to
   shoot. You're disciplined, but there are times . . .'
'Yeah, times when we are all too human.'
The emotions were still strong. His eyes were stinging. Graham took a tissue and
   blew his nose. 'This ain't easy, is it?'
'No, it's not, but you're doing well.'
'Never really said much about Geordie to anyone, and I feel I want to now. I want
   you to know him. He was important to me, all those years ago, but I said to
   myself and to him – just before he died – "I won't forget you, Geordie, I won't
   ever forget you".'
'And you kept your promise.'
'Yeah. He was a mate, more than a mate. We were buddies and often we'd be
   together in a vehicle, but somehow we weren't that day. I don't know why.
   We should have been together, dead or alive . . .'
'Together, dead or alive . . .' Oliver stayed with the focus Graham had reached,
   and waited.
'Could have been me, maybe should have been me . . .' Graham lapsed into silence.
Oliver respected the short silence that followed after responding with 'could have,
   maybe should have been you . . .'
'It's part of it, wondering, why you're alive, and someone else isn't. Yet you have
   to cope, move on. He was dead, I was alive. They told me to accept it, that was
   how it was. I wanted to make sense of it. They said you couldn't, no point in
   trying, that was how it was.' He paused. 'And you do accept it. And now, well,
   now I wonder.'
'Now you wonder, now you need to make sense of it?'
'If I'd died and he was alive, you know, maybe he'd be making a better job of civilian life than me. I don't know, I think he would have done better.'

The temptation was always to say no, to reassure, but the reality was that Graham had his thoughts and Oliver was there to empathise. 'That's a tough one, thinking he might have done better at civilian life.'

Graham nodded, tight-lipped once more. 'His family came from Newcastle, that's why we called him Geordie. Real name was Chris, Chris Marriott. I went to his funeral, of course.' He shook his head. 'I tried to tell his parents how great a lad their son was, said a few words at the funeral. Kept in touch with them for a few years but somehow things drifted. Feel bad about that. Feel I let Geordie down, somehow.' Graham paused.

'Feel like you let him down by losing contact.'

'But life goes on, new experiences, new challenges, but I never have forgotten him. Always one for a joke, always had a fag spare, would have given you the shirt off his back if you asked for it.' Graham was shaking his head and had closed his eyes. 'And he was one for the women, just had that something. It wasn't that he was particularly good looking, but he just had a way about him. Maybe it was the accent, I think that helped, but you could never keep track of the women in his life.' Graham was smiling.

'Some good memories as well, yeah?'

Graham nodded. 'Yeah. Poor bastard, everything to live for, whole life ahead of him, and then one bomb and it was all over. He was one of those people you really had to like, and somehow, well, we clicked. Good times.' Another wave of emotion and Graham closed his eyes, fighting it back.

The atmosphere in the room had grown progressively quieter and more intense. Oliver was aware that he wasn't saying much, but it wasn't a session that needed him to speak. Graham was the one who needed to talk. For Oliver the important thing was to be there, be attentive, listen, empathise, be present and respectful towards what Graham was saying and experiencing, and not get in the way but let his process take him where he needed to go.

Graham had pursed his lips and was blowing air out. 'And there's many more incidents like that though none quite the same, nothing is quite the same as that first death of a buddy.' He paused. 'But that was a long time ago. And there were other tragedies in Northern Ireland. I honestly believe we were trying to do a job, trying to keep two communities apart from each other, but I can see now that there was a lot of politics. At the time, well, you didn't think like that. You were given orders, given tasks to perform and you got on with it ... Yeah, you got on with it.'

'Mhmm, you couldn't see the politics at the time, but now ...'

'... now there's no doubt in my mind that things were manipulated, and it was a war. Everyone avoided using the word, but it was war on the streets. And it was vicious. There were some nasty things done on both sides, and for what? In the name of religion? Bullshit. Just people who wanted to hurt and kill, and religion was a convenient cause. I don't know if it's fear or what it is, but from generation to generation people are conditioned into bigotry and hatred. Not everyone, not everyone, there were those trying to build bridges across the communities, and maybe things are changing now, but I don't know. There is still so much terrorising, and drugs are everywhere. You don't read about it much in the papers, but there's still a lot of nasty things happening. War on terror? There's still terror on the streets and in those estates. What do we do about terror? We bomb the Iraqis. Poor bastards. But you're given a job, and you do it. That's how it is.'

Oliver nodded. 'A time of your life that made a deep impression on you, affected you in many ways, so many thoughts, feelings, memories.' He spoke deliberately, not wanting to sound as though he was trying to tie all that Graham had said up into some neat bundle. It wasn't. It was messy and painful, and not neat. 'A messy, painful business.'

Should Oliver have empathised more directly with what Graham was saying, and the way his thoughts had developed, or was a more general empathy more appropriate? Is Oliver uncomfortable empathising with Graham's views and is that preventing a more precise empathic response?

'Yeah. Gave me the taste of death, made me see another world, one that, well, you see stuff on TV and in films, but that's bullshit. Sixty seconds of sanitised film that's shown again and again. I've heard the screams, the real screams, seen the despair and the hatred in people's eyes. I've seen a young girl tarred and feathered, seen what women can do to another woman.' Graham shook his head. 'And I know why you shoot to kill. To stop the killing, to take someone out, but there are always others to replace them.'

'I can't know what it was like, but listening to you speak I grow cold, a creeping coldness, and a sense of despair, and a horror that you had to witness what you witnessed.'

'It should affect people like that. And I appreciate you being honest. You weren't there, though I don't know anything about you, and maybe you have had similar experiences, I don't know.'

'No, I was never in the military, and no, I haven't faced the kind of events that you have had to face, and I listen to what you have to say and I try to understand what it is like for you, as you sit here, describing what you have seen, and what you have experienced. And I am horrified by what people do to one another, but I have only watched TV and read about it. You have been there, and in some strange way it feels very humbling to hear you speak; you bring me closer to a world that is beyond my experience. It can only affect me and I hope make me more sensitive as a result.'

'Like I said, what you see on TV is nothing, most of the time it's a joke. They're scared of showing us the truth. A bit more reality and maybe things might be different. I don't know.'

'And I guess I'd feel different too.'

'You know, whilst it is about seeing bodies broken and tortured, it isn't that so much as the sense that it was another human-being that did it. And I'm a human-being. Pain inflicted very often by men – and I am a man. And I want to believe I am different, but I know, I know that I can strike out if I am hurt and angry, and could I do the same? I like to think not, but there have been times when I have doubted that. I feel as though we are a disciplined army, and I know that stuff has come to light in Iraq that really does not make us look good, and I can imagine things happening. On the whole, there is a lot of discipline, but people break under pressure and need to release what builds up inside them. You see your mate gunned down beside you, or see someone from your regiment being dragged around behind a truck, you're human, you want to fight back, you want to get someone, and it can be pretty ugly. War is ugly. Brings out the best, some say, and it brings out the worst. And in the heat of battle the line between them can get very blurred. You have to keep your discipline, that's the difference between living, and dying.' Graham spoke very slowly and deliberately, the words, each word, carried power and made an impression.

Oliver was aware of sitting and feeling quite overwhelmed by all that Graham had been saying. He felt full, as though Graham had somehow filled him up with experiences, and yet he knew that in reality Graham had shared very little, but he had spoken with such an intensity, that he had made a huge impact. Oliver felt alert and yet strangely drained. He had been listening with such concentration for most of the session, saying very little, but being there, hoping to convey his acceptance of Graham and of what he was saying. He didn't feel he had offered much verbal empathy, but that wasn't always appropriate in his view when someone needed to talk at length. Attention, facial expression, posture could all convey what was needed for the interaction to have therapeutic value.

'What you say leaves me with so many different thoughts and feelings, but most of all a sense of wanting to ask, "what about you? How have you coped? Where are you in yourself in sharing something of your past experiences?"'

Graham tightened his lips and shook his head, his expression was grim. 'How do you live with a head full of memories like I have?'

'I guess painfully, minute to minute, maybe second by second, finding your way through it all.'

Graham took a deep breath and nodded. 'Thank you. Yes, that is how it is at the moment. And there are times when you can forget, when you lose yourself in something that you are doing, or you have a few extra beers, you know?'

'I can only imagine.'

'But it is short-lived. The pain is always there. Something gets to you, gets into your very soul. You can't see life like others do, it's hard to smile and laugh, really smile and laugh. You do, everyone does. You work hard, you play hard. But looking back now, well, it's sort of unreal, somehow, an escape. I haven't laughed like that for a while now. Certainly not since leaving the army. It robs you of something, Oliver, and I feel as though I am missing something of myself.'

'No laughter, no smiles, constant pain and it's as if some part of you has gone missing.'

'Yeah, gone walkabout . . .'

'Part of you has gone walkabout.'

'Yeah.' Graham sighed. He lapsed into silence, staring ahead, feeling and not feeling. He hadn't said much, not really, but had he said enough? He knew there was so much to tell, but he would be weeks if he did that and he wasn't prepared to do that. It did feel good to have spoken about some of the events though, and it was different talking to Oliver. He listened, really listened, and didn't try and minimise it. He seemed to accept it and be affected by it. Graham needed that. He needed to know that events in his life did affect people. But he still didn't know what to do. It wasn't as though his experiences in Northern Ireland were the ones that woke him in the night, but they were his first experiences of vicious, human violence. He sat in his own thoughts.

Oliver remains silent, not wishing to disturb Graham as he sits, clearly engaging with his own internal thought processes. He knows that he cannot really imagine what it must be like to have your best mate die in pain in your arms, his body shattered and shredded by shrapnel, and of seeing body parts after a bombing. He knows he has nothing to offer Graham but himself as a fellow human-being, ready and willing to listen and, as best he can, share his human response to the inhuman actions described. But was it inhuman? We like to say that extreme violence is inhuman, but it is human-beings that do it, and therefore it is something that human-beings have the capacity to do to each other. The hard reality is that it is all too human, and this leaves Oliver wondering at what, in different circumstances, and given different conditioning, he might have been capable of. He hopes that he would not be able to inflict violence on others, but the truth is, the hard truth is, that he does not know. He just hopes that it is something he would be incapable of, but he cannot be sure. He realises he wants to explore this in supervision. He has drifted into his own thoughts and away from Graham; he brings himself back.

Graham was continuing. 'You keep going, but it's an effort, it is at the moment. I guess in the army you had each other, there was a culture of getting on with it, you have things you had to do. But now, well, I feel much more isolated, and, well, there's a choice not to do things. You can't choose not to do things in the army. I feel like I've shut down inside, and yet I haven't. It feels sometimes like I'm exhausted with it all, utterly, utterly exhausted.'

Oliver responded, sensing the tiredness in Graham's voice, 'shut down, overwhelmed by it all and, yeah, tired and utterly exhausted with it.'

Graham nodded. 'I guess it's no wonder I'm not coping too well at the moment.'

'Mhmm, hard to feel like you're coping?'

'I'm not, but I can't seem to be any different.'

'Maybe you need to be as you are, maybe this is part of the healing process, time to stop and lick your wounds, as it were.'

Not an empathic response. Oliver has offered an explanation or interpretation of what Graham is experiencing. Oliver has moved away from person-centred practice. A simple empathic, 'mhmm, feels like you just can't be any different' would have sufficed. However, what Oliver says resonates with Graham. It might be argued that the way Oliver is with Graham is more empathic to Graham's style and way of being, or is it a collusion with some kind of man-to-man dynamic which avoids the awkwardness and discomfort that might arise from a different style of response?

Graham heard what Oliver was saying. It made sense. He didn't like it, went against the grain, but he felt he had no choice. He simply did not have the energy to do anything.

'You think I should accept it? That feels hard. I should be fighting it, pushing myself.'

'You feel that strongly, hard to accept, you should be pushing, fighting?'

'To accept it would be to give up, I can't do that.'

'Accepting is giving up, that's what it means to you . . . ?' Oliver had intended to empathise with the "I can't do that", but Graham was speaking.

'Yes, and I can't do that, but I can't seem to push myself. I feel exhausted just sitting here.'

'You've done a lot of work today, Graham, talked about some really important and significant experiences.'

'And I've only scratched the surface, and that's . . .' he sighed, 'that's not very encouraging'.

'That you feel like this after only scratching the surface?'

'Yes, there's so much more.' Graham looked away, his mind had drifted to Bosnia, the ethnic cleansing, the rape camps, the mass graves, death all around.

'Mhmm, so much more.'

'Will it help?'

'I believe so.'

Graham looked searchingly towards Oliver. Deep down he knew he had to talk, but it would mean filling Oliver's head with the shit in his own and he wasn't sure that he wanted to do that to him. Oliver was obviously trained, and a professional, but not to see what he had seen, or hear what he had heard, surely. You had to have a military training to cope with that. Crazy thought, he thought to himself. Here am I, having had a military training, and I'm the one needing to talk about it.

'You want to hear?' Graham looked at Oliver. It was a crucial moment.

Oliver felt a slight smile inside himself, he recognised the moment, and he also felt a certain grimness inside himself, sensing he was about to say he wanted to hear what Graham needed to say, whilst aware that part of him would rather he didn't. 'I want to help and, yes, I want to hear, even if I may feel myself recoiling from something you say, but that doesn't mean I don't want to hear and understand what you've experienced. I'm prepared to make that journey with you, Graham. I can't take away memories, but there are ways that people discover to manage them. You managed them in the military, but they've caught up with you now, and maybe new ways are required, or maybe the act of telling your story, of feeling it heard and validated in some way, will make enough difference.' Oliver felt like he had perhaps said too much, but he knew he needed to communicate something of his thoughts and hopes for what he could offer. It felt like a critical moment in the counselling process. He knew he must trust Graham to make his choice. He would either feel ready to continue, or would seek other ways of trying to deal with the effects of his military career.

'I came wanting answers, expecting you to "do something", to, I don't know, I'm not sure what I was thinking, but maybe to put me through some psychological process that would make me feel myself again. But that isn't the way, is it?'

'I don't know what will emerge. I am only beginning to sense the you that is coming into this process. I don't know what "you" will come out of it.'

'Neither do I. But it feels like I have no choice. I don't want pills. I want to get back into life, my job, family, all the things that are important to me. But it's like the past is a barrier, an obstacle, and I can't push it out of the way.'

'You feel like you should push it out of the way?'

'Yes, yes I do, and I know that I can't. And it feels like it's growing, getting bigger, and that perhaps talking about things adds to it, and I'm not sure whether that will just make it worse.'

'If I talk about it, will it get worse, will that obstacle, that barrier grow and separate me even more from the important things in my life – job, family . . . ?'

Oliver has switched to speaking in the first person, putting into words what Graham is pondering, and in the words that Graham would have been thinking about it. This can be a powerful form of empathy. It proves facilitative.

'I've faced a few enemies in my life.' Graham drew a deep breath and let the air out slowly. 'Now I have to face myself, my past.'

'Yes.' Oliver didn't feel he had much to add. The simple affirmation felt appropriate, leaving Graham with his insight on his situation.

The session drew to a close. It felt like a natural ending and Graham somehow felt more clear in himself. It wasn't that he had answers, but he did have a kind of knowing that he had to push on with the counselling, that he had to deal with his past and with how it was affecting him. He didn't quite know what that meant, or what it would mean for him in the future. He knew part of him wanted to batten down the hatches, as it were, and just try and get on with things, but he also knew that he had been doing that in recent weeks and months, and it hadn't worked. He had tried to keep going, but he'd had to stop. Now he had to do what was necessary to get himself going again. Well, that's what he would do, however long it took. But he also knew that he did need to get back to work. Whilst his wife worked and they could get by for a while, he knew he needed to get himself working. But he had to find some strength for that from somewhere. He knew he had a lot to think about.

Oliver returned to the counselling room after Graham had left. He knew he had no magic wand to turn around the effects of Graham's experience in a few weeks, in a few sessions of therapy, but he felt confident that he could make a start, begin a process with Graham, maybe help him get back to work and then refer him on for longer term therapy if he felt he wanted it. There were no guarantees that Graham would. He could only take it week by week, maintain the therapeutic conditions, and allow Graham's actualising tendency to … he always struggled with the words to describe the process. It was growth, development, adaptation, and yet somehow there was something simple at the heart of all the complexity, the simplicity of learning to be yourself, of accepting who you are, what you are. He'd had his own barriers to this. But he had discovered that they existed because he had separated off aspects of himself from his normal, everyday awareness. Only by reintegrating with these separated parts of himself had he begun to dissolve his barriers.

Yes, like standing on a path with a rock blocking your way, you have to discover the rocks in yourself, and then you realise that you are the rock in front of you, and then, slowly, painfully, comes the realisation that as you accept this, and begin to process what created it, it can begin to feel less solid. You begin to become less of an obstacle to yourself, see beyond the rock in yourself and start to tread the path that lies beyond it as the rock-like obstacles in yourself begin to erode away. Oliver believed that therapeutic relationship based on the values and principles of person-centred working would enable the rocks within Graham to erode and he would find a way forward that was right for him.

Points for discussion

- What feelings and thoughts has this counselling session left you with?
- Critically evaluate Oliver's application of the person-centred approach.
- What is the quality of your empathy for Graham? Define for yourself, and in your own words, the impressions that Graham is making on you.
- Can you identify any particularly critical or significant moments in the counselling session, and, if so, what made them important?
- How do you sense Graham's view of Oliver to be at the end of this session? Do you think it has changed and, if so, why and how?
- How do you respond to Oliver's thoughts after the session? Is this how you see the process? How would you describe it with a metaphor of your own?
- Write notes for this session.

CHAPTER 12

Counselling session 3: a positive shift as Graham releases feelings from his experiences in Bosnia

Oliver sat in the counselling room at the surgery, watching the rain stream-
ing down against the window. Not a very pleasant day, he thought.
He'd already had one client not attend without word and wondered whether
the weather had played a part in that decision. It was now 3 pm and time
for Graham. He got up and headed out to the waiting room just in time to see
Graham coming through the door.

'Hello Graham, come on through.'

'Thanks. It's not nice out there. I've only walked from the car park but that was
enough to get wet.'

They went into the counselling room, Graham hanging his damp coat up on the
hook behind the door.

Oliver was aware that he had no idea what Graham would want to talk about.
A week had passed between sessions and whilst, for him, there was a sense of
continuing from the previous session, he was aware that for Graham, as for
any client, the process did not stop when they left the room. One thing Oliver
was sure of was that Graham was not a person who would have his hour with
the counsellor, walk away and forget it until the next week. The effects of his
past were too present for him. He felt sure that Graham would have thought
about what he wanted to talk about today and he was not going to undermine this by directing him on to some theme, or focusing him back on the previous session.

The essential non-directive nature of person-centred therapy is very much
at the core of the approach. Whilst it is not mentioned as a 'core condition' it
is nevertheless a significant feature of the approach, and something that dif-
ferentiates it from other therapeutic approaches. Indeed, writing in 1942,
Rogers began to contrast directive and non-directive approaches, compar-
ing a short number of interviews but demonstrating that directive therapy
involved the directive therapists using almost six times the number of words

used as the non-directive therapists. His emphasis on the value and effectiveness of non-directive nature of therapy evolved into a realisation that it was the quality of the relationship that was more important than any techniques that a therapist might employ (Kirschenbaum and Henderson, 1990 citing Rogers, 1942).

'How do you want to use the time today, Graham?'

'You know, I've been thinking a lot this week, and it's strange, it has felt a little different, like I'm doing the thinking rather than thoughts imposing themselves on me. At least, in relation to some things.'

'Mhmm, more in control of your thinking?' Oliver wasn't sure if that was quite what Graham was saying so his response had a questioning tone to it.

'Yes, I think so, but I could be fooling myself. I do realise that I am my own obstacle. It's not the events of the past that are in the way, it's me, how I've been affected. Something I hadn't really thought about, in fact it seems that coming here is making me think, and yet I always saw myself as someone who did think, but didn't feel. It's strange, and hard to really describe.'

'Let's see if I can understand what you mean. It's like you have always seen yourself as a thinking person, rather than a feeling person, but somehow the nature of your thinking – towards the past and towards yourself – has changed in some way, but that actual change is hard to describe.'

'Mmm. Something like that, yes.' Graham looked thoughtful and frowned. 'It's strange.' He shook his head. 'You think you're so in control, so strong, so able to cope with anything, because you have coped with anything, and then ...' He took a deep breath and eased back into the seat, '... and then you find yourself having to be here, no disrespect to you, but having to talk to a counsellor, something I'd never have believed I'd have needed.' He paused, Oliver was about to respond, but Graham continued. 'But I am here, and I do need this, and part of me still wants to leave here and not deal with any of it.'

'You've had a very controlling career, and being here is such a contrast to that and yes, part of you wants to be out that door and back in control.'

'Yes. You say "a very controlling career", and you are right, in many ways, but the things that happened I had no control over, not really. OK, we would be involved in planned operations, and yes, it was all thought through, but then when things started you could be thinking on your feet. And there would be times when you knew you were reacting, or responding to someone else's reaction. You stayed disciplined, or you tried to, but there was always the unexpected, things that you couldn't prepare yourself for.' Graham coughed. It sounded to Oliver as though Graham's voice had become a little weaker.

'The unexpected.' He didn't say anything more, he sensed that what Graham had said had put him in touch with a memory and he didn't want to disturb that.

'And you react differently to situations, and you're surprised at the reaction.' He frowned and stared down to the right of Graham. 'Things were bad in Northern Ireland, yes, they were, and maybe because it was my first tour, and my first experience of death first hand, it stays with me in some way. But it was worse in Bosnia.' Graham went quiet and swallowed. 'I hate that phrase, "ethnic cleansing", it sounds so sanitised. I don't know who came up with it but they should be fucking shot. I know what it means. I've seen the effects. There is nothing sanitary about it, nothing cleansing, just people being destroyed by any means, utter carnage.' He went quiet again.

Oliver did not respond, it did not feel necessary. He respected the silence and the pace at which Graham was speaking. It felt more appropriate to allow him to continue to engage with his own flow of thoughts, feelings and memories than to draw him into a verbal interaction.

By not responding, Graham is given the space to remain with his thoughts and feelings. Oliver maintains his attention and his heartfelt sense of warm acceptance for Graham, and waits to see what direction he wants to take the session in after connecting with memories from Bosnia.

Graham was aware of Oliver, and sensed his attention, but his own attention was much more on the images and the sounds in his head.

'What's worse? Being confronted with the living, or with the dead?' Graham had looked up.

Oliver had no idea what train of thought had brought Graham to this comment, but he kept his response simple, and direct, as it seemed a direct question. 'I don't know.'

Graham heard the response and it matched his own thinking. He didn't know either. It encouraged him to continue. 'I've seen mass graves, and I've seen people brutalised. I've looked into their eyes, eyes that have witnessed horrors that no eyes should have seen. Dead eyes in which the only sense of life is fear.'

Oliver maintained his silence, listening with every fibre of his being to what Graham was saying, striving to be totally present as a human-being as he continued to speak.

Graham was shaking his head, his lips tight, his face had paled. He'd never forget the smell. The scene was bad enough, the bodies, bloodied and mutilated, piled up and rotting, but it was the smell that haunted him . . .

Silence.

Oliver sat, no idea what Graham was re-living, and not wishing to intrude on his process and focus. He believed, wholeheartedly, that there were times when the presence of another was enough for therapeutic effect. Graham was re-living his experiences in the presence of another person and for Oliver there was a belief that there was a healing possibility in that process. Maybe not immediately, maybe not for a long time, but for another person to stay with you as you re-connected with past traumas, to offer you attention, to be that person to stop the other feeling alone with their memories, somehow in that process there was a therapeutic possibility.

Graham's eyes began to water. He was back with the faces of the women who had been abandoned at the rape camp that they had come across, and quite unexpectedly. 'None of us had been prepared for it. No one knew what to do. Fear, pain, anguish, terror, moanings and whimperings, raw sounds that spoke the language of man's potential to inflict sexual brutality and savagery on women, and these had been Muslim women, rounded up, their husbands and sons and fathers taken away, and probably all shot – or worse.'

He took a short sharp breath and let it out. He didn't want the emotion to get the better of him, not in front of a man, but his throat was burning. Another short sharp intake and out-take of breath.

Oliver was aware of Graham's breathing and the water in his eyes. He saw a tear run down his cheek, and another. 'Let it out, Graham, it's safe here.'

Graham knew he couldn't afford tears for his comrades in arms, you didn't shed tears, but the civilians, the victims, the women, he felt a surge of emotion running up from his stomach and a wave of tears filled his eyes. He swallowed but his throat was dry. He closed his eyes and sent tears running down his face. He screwed his eyes up as another wave of emotion, of pain, tore from his solar plexus area up through his heart and throat and into his eyes. He was shaking his head now. He swallowed, he was breathing now in short sharp breaths, he opened his mouth to speak, but there were no words to say. Another wave of pain and anguish, and feelings of utter helplessness, the feelings of standing there, in that camp, not knowing what to do.

Graham opened his eyes and looked at Oliver. 'They thought we were going to rape them as well. Because we were soldiers, because we were men. Young girls, women, their faces, their torn clothes, but worst of all was their eyes. Terror.' Another deep breath. 'We managed to communicate to them who we were, that we were not there to hurt them, but to set them free – "set them free!" – what the hell does that mean? Well, at least they were free, but I can only imagine that they will never really be free.' He swallowed and reached for the glass of water on the table. He returned the glass and eased back into the chair, closing his eyes again as he did so.

'Yeah, never be free of . . .'

'We did what we could, and we radioed for medical support. We stayed in the area a while, and some were detailed to remain behind, but I was among those that had to move out and continue on.' Another wave of emotion hit him as he thought about something else he had come across, a young woman hanging from a tree, a woman who had taken her own life rather than be caught. It was an image that he knew had got into the press and had appeared in the newspapers. But he had seen it for real, seen her hanging there.

'The women were killing themselves to avoid being caught.'

Oliver nodded, his own memories were stirring now.

'You may have seen a photo in the papers. I saw it for real.'

Oliver had seen that photo and it had made a deep impression on him at the time, and he felt a surge of emotion inside himself and his own eyes watering. Yes, he had cried when he had seen that photo, and now he cried again.

'Yes,' he swallowed, 'yes, I know the one you mean.'

'There's nothing to say, is there?' It was Graham who spoke.

'Nothing, and everything', was Oliver's response, 'nothing and everything.'

The two men lapsed into a silence, a mutual moment of being, each touched by the pain of the other written in their eyes. And yet amidst the emotion was a calmness, a stillness as the pain eased, yet it was fleeting, and was gone. Neither spoke of it, but each had felt its presence. It made a deep impression on Graham, and as it faded he found himself thinking again of the piles of corpses he'd witnessed.

> There is almost a role reversal as Oliver's own emotions rise to the surface. In that moment, in the context of what was being re-lived, that is acceptable. Both men are being congruent, expressing feelings over a commonly experienced event. It is OK for counsellors to show their feelings and to cry with a client, so long as it is not something they make a habit of. But situations do arise that demand it of the counsellor. Something is said, the feelings arise, the eyes water, tears flow. But even in that moment the counsellor will be striving to maintain contact with the client, and maintain their flow of empathic sensitivity to what the client is experiencing and communicating.

It was Graham who spoke first. 'I think I'd buried and locked up my feelings towards those women, Oliver, until now. The images that have been most present were of the dead bodies in the mass graves, and the smell . . . It's a smell that haunts you, a smell of death that goes beyond the smell of a rotting corpse.'

'Buried under the corpses.' Oliver's response had been utterly instinctive, without any thought, and the moment he heard the words he wondered if they were right, and yet somehow they seemed exactly right.

'Yeah, something like that.' Graham blew out a long breath. 'I feel weird, but I feel strangely more in touch with myself.'

'More in touch with . . . feelings?'

Graham nodded. He took another breath and again blew the air out slowly.

'The woman who hung herself, she wasn't the only one, she would have been living her life, plans for her future, family maybe, who knows. And then . . .' Graham shook his head. 'Whatever state of mind must she have been in? Whatever would she have been feeling, her world shattered, ripped apart, running to get away, terror at what men would do to her.'

At what men would do to her. Oliver felt very aware of being a man himself and he knew how he himself had wrestled with his identity as a man given the actions that men take towards women. He had written a poem many years before as part of his own process. He made a note to look it out when he got home.

'It's awful, just trying to imagine, the terror at what the men would do to her.' Oliver was aware of the strength of his own feelings and how they threatened to distance him from Graham's world of experience which would not be the same, however much there might be similarities. His feelings were at risk of obscuring his sensitivity towards those of Graham. He made a conscious effort to bring his focus back on to Graham.

'Why didn't we do something sooner? Why do we always wait until it is too late in these situations? Every time we delay, not wanting to interfere in a country's internal affairs. Wasn't it Nero who was supposed to have played the fiddle while Rome burned? When you see the faces, when you look into the eyes, when you've seen the bodies piled high, and smelt death and terror ... Why do we wait?'

'Yeah, why do we wait ... ?'

'We messed up in Bosnia, big time. Thousands were killed and brutalised, and it could have been avoided. We faffed about. I know, I'm sure people had the best of intentions, but the reality is we balls'd it up, big time. When will we give the UN an army and pass international laws to give it the power to not just keep peace, but be able to fight for that peace?'

Oliver was aware that the conversation had moved away from feelings, into thoughts and speculations. He respected Graham's shift of emphasis. Graham needed to air his views, maybe give himself respite from the emotion, maybe provide a focus to vent his frustration. He wasn't going to direct Graham back. He needed to say what he was saying, these were clearly important thoughts for him. 'A quicker and different response when the situation is developing?'

'We were too late. We could have stopped it. I have no doubt about that. All that suffering.' He shook his head.

'Yeah, all that suffering ...'

'Leaves me angry, fucking angry.'

'Angry towards?'

'Governments, politicians. The bastards in Serbia, Croatia, all over the region, that encouraged it all. And they still haven't got Karodicz.'

Oliver felt that probably there was a lot more anger in Graham, but it hadn't really broken into his awareness, not yet. He wasn't going to push it, maybe there was a need for more pain and sadness to emerge before then? He empathised with what Graham was telling him.

'You feel a lot of anger towards a lot of people.'

'At least we were a bit quicker in Kosovo, had time there as well, and we did learn from Bosnia. Why can't people put the past aside?'

'Why can't people in these places forgive and forget, do you mean?'

'Yes, and I know they can't, and maybe I wouldn't be able to either. Oh, I don't know.'

Time was passing, there were ten minutes left of the session. Graham noticed Oliver glance at the clock. 'How're we doing?'

'Fine, ten minutes left.'

'OK. It's been quite a session, and I feel wiped out, I have to say, and my feelings are still close.'

'You've burned up a lot of emotional energy this afternoon.'

'I needed to. I kind of knew before I came today that I was going to have to touch into some of this stuff. It's strange, but the images I have in the night are dead bodies, and that smell. It never goes away, at least it does, but it's kind of hovering close by, and I smell it in the night. I wake up, sweating, really restless.

Angela's really good. I haven't told her much about it. Don't want her to have to carry it as well. She tries to get me to talk to her sometimes, but I don't. Usually have a drink. Doesn't help always but it sort of feels like the thing to do.' Graham paused. 'Do you think I'll ever lose that smell?'

'I can't say, Graham. Smell is one of the most powerful of senses, can take us back into memories so fast. And in any moment of trauma the senses seem to be more alert and what we sense is imprinted more deeply, more acutely, and maybe in a different way, hence people experience forms of traumatic shock.'

'The doctor mentioned that. I guess I've experienced enough traumatising shocks to have that, but you don't think about it, not at the time. And maybe it isn't always traumatising, you've got used to it. And then something happens, and then it's different. Geordie. The bodies, and the eyes of those women,' he shook his head. 'You do what you have to do, but sometimes you can feel in a daze. You try not to be, and usually you're sharp, but sometimes, just sometimes you drift, you wonder – those are dangerous moments. You have to pull yourself together. It's what you do, you're part of a group, a team, you get on with it, you know, and you can, you do. And of course at home it gets to you. I'd have sleepless night at home before I left the army. But somehow still being part of it helped. But now, now it feels like I'm on my own.'

'No longer part of the team, part of the Regiment. Feels more like you're on your own.'

Oliver has shown only partial empathy, highlighting one aspect of what Graham has been saying. It is a difficult situation when a client says a number of things. Do you respond with a general empathic comment, or respond to the last thing mentioned to acknowledge where the client's process has brought them so they can then continue, or do you try to summarise all that has been said? And if you spend too long trying to decide the moment has past, spontaneity is lost, the flow is disturbed. The decision is a mix of instinct and experience, a kind of sensing of what is needed, but the therapist may not always choose the most facilitative or therapeutically valuable response.

The Regiment. It had been his family. It still meant a lot for him and yet . . . 'Yes. Been back for a reunion. I don't know if that was a good thing or not. But it was my family, you know, I mean, you get so close to people. Yes, I love my wife and children, but it's different. You know you are facing life or death situations. It's different. You bond in a different way.'

'Bond in a different way?'

'Hard to explain. You just do. It's like it's of a different order, somehow. There's no doubt, total trust – there has to be. Yeah, and belief, self-belief and belief in those around you. You have to have belief to go into combat – you have to.'

'That belief is so crucial.' Oliver nodded slowly.

'And it's real, so fucking real, closer than family.' Graham looked at Oliver.

'So real and so much closer.' Oliver maintained the eye contact.

'In a way it was, but it also felt unreal, at least, now it does, and yet it doesn't. But it doesn't exist in civilian life. When I went back it was like I'd moved on, and yet somehow I hadn't. I still haven't really got used to civilian life, and I wonder sometimes if I ever will. Not surprised people leaving the military end up in security jobs.'

'Something about security jobs?'

'Team work, discipline, routine, clarity.'

'Mhmm.'

'I don't know. I feel like I've started something now, here, with you, and I don't know what will happen, but I did need to talk and feel, like I have today and last week. I think it's going to help me come alive again. Does that sound strange?'

'No, not to me, but it sounds like it might for you?'

'I'm actually not too sure what it means to be alive, I mean, really alive, except, well, in the army, training, combat, yes, you were alive then, at least you were sharp, focused, and yet what I have found already coming here is a sense that maybe in that there was something missing, something that couldn't be present because it would have got in the way.' He paused before continuing. 'I think I've been living some other kind of life, like I think I said before, not really being able to smile, really smile, really feel happy. It's like the edge is always taken off things.' Graham thought to himself and he found himself thinking that he only really laughed when he'd had a few beers. And even then, that didn't always work. Sometimes he simply felt depressed.

'Mhmm, edge taken off so you can't really smile or really feel happy.'

'Maybe that's what I need to do, learn to smile, try and find those feelings, but I wonder if I ever will. I've seen too much, Oliver, of the darker side of humanity. I feel like damaged goods, here.'

Oliver nodded, 'damaged by the darker side, you mean?'

Graham stopped as a thought struck him, and powerfully so. It was a "stop the world moment". 'Yes, and it's not the bodies or the faces of the women that damaged me, they were the effects. The real damage was done by the fucking bastards that perpetrated it all. They are the ones, and I owe it to those women to not let those fucking bastards keep me down.' He was looking at Oliver, 'that's it, isn't it, the images in my head are those of the innocents. I owe it to them to get on with my life, not to forget, or to belittle their suffering . . .'

'. . . to live your life in spite of the things that you have witnessed, that you know happen and still happen in parts of the world.' Oliver felt as though he had come in too quickly, perhaps robbing Graham of his own words. He bit his lip. 'Sorry, I think I cut across you.'

'It's OK. I think today has helped me to lift the lid a little and let the pressure out. I guess I need to ensure I don't clamp it back down again.'

Oliver nodded. 'And I don't want to lose sight of the comment you made just now about identifying the real cause of the images in your head, the, as you say, "fucking bastards that perpetrated it".'

'I've been affected, yes, maybe traumatised, by the effects of their actions. I don't imagine the images will go away. But somehow, something has shifted a little inside me. I can't really define it, but there is a difference. It's time I headed off. Thanks for this afternoon. Once again, much to go away and think about. This isn't easy, but it feels really helpful. Thanks.' Graham offered his hand, Oliver took it.

'Counselling isn't easy, it isn't the "soft option" some think. I'm pleased you are experiencing benefit from this. Take care of yourself, you may feel quite disorientated having engaged with such powerful feelings. You may want to give yourself a quiet time to just bring yourself back together, as it were. The noise of the world can sometimes seem quite harsh after this kind of session.'

Graham nodded. 'Yes, I felt that last time, and I'm sure it'll be the same this week as well. He took his coat and headed out through the door. He noted immediately that the noise of the full waiting room seemed strangely loud and overwhelming. It was still raining. He needed quiet to just be with his thoughts.

Points for discussion

- How has the session affected you? What made the greatest impression, and why?
- What would you identify as being your greatest challenge to working with Graham?
- How might you have responded differently from Oliver during the session, and why, and how would you justify it from a person-centred perspective?
- Think of the differences as to how a male and female counsellor might react to Graham's description of his Bosnia experience.
- Do you believe that there are times when the presence of the counsellor is enough to maintain a therapeutic relationship?
- Evaluate the accuracy of Oliver's empathic responding. How has he communicated the 'core conditions'? Give examples.
- Write notes for this session.

* * *

That evening Graham looked out the poem that he had written. In doing so another one fell out of the file, one he had forgotten about. He'd written it a little after the fall of the Berlin Wall, at around the time of the struggle in Rumania to overthrow the regime that was in power – Christmas 1989. He found himself reading it before the one he had been looking for.

Freedom's Cost

Shattered forms are strewn across the darkened streets of pain
Where hope was born had died was born to live in hearts again.
Tortured bodies buried, so many barbed wire bound,
A legacy of evil that for too long did abound.

Visions of a future time where freedom's bell would ring
Had touched the minds of many, but the struggle it would bring
Would test the souls of those who stood to fight for what was good,
The final freedom they attained was written in their blood.

Nothing True or Real is ever gained without a cost,
And all our strivings that we make for freedom are not lost.
The will that drives the spirit into greater liberty
Lies at the heart of that great Life we call humanity.

After a period of reflection, and wondering whether he should share it with Graham, and deciding not to, he picked up the second poem, the one that he had been reminded of during the session.

Eyes of Wonder

Eyes of wonder, peace and charm.
A new born babe upon my arm.
Little fingers clutching out,
Explores the world around about.
Majestic jewel, creation's glory
Enters the eternal story
And takes her place within a world
With bright blue eyes and gold hair curled

And yet this babe, this child to be,
Her eyes so bright, who smiles at me;
Will she still shine when men have done
To womanhood . . . They have their fun
And leave a trail of pain and fears
Oblivious to her sobs and tears.
Expect, demand is all they know;
A woman's place, to take below.

Dear God, when will we men begin
To cast aside this dreadful sin
And realise a woman's place
Beside us in the human race.
We wouldn't dream of doing harm
To eyes of wonder, peace and charm.

CHAPTER 13

Supervision session 1: pain and compassion

'So, you said at the start of the session you wanted some time to talk about your new client.' Jean had been supervising Oliver for three years and she valued their sessions as he really was passionate about his work. She appreciated that quality and had voiced it to him in the past.

'Victim of warfare. But on the military side. His name's Graham, had 20 years in the army, served in various places – he's talked about Northern Ireland and Bosnia. He's off work, clearly stressed, head full of traumatic memories, feelings locked up but now being expressed, and he's really using the counselling. And it's throwing up issues for me, as well.'

'So, where do you want to start?'

'He's talked about being in Northern Ireland and holding his best mate in his arms as he died after being blown up. He's talked of his despair at the inhumanity he has witnessed, and of the kind of things that happened over there. That was in the second session. In the last session he talked about Bosnia, about the images of dead bodies, and of entering one of the rape camps and how it affected him. He talked about being a man and a soldier and how the women feared them, thinking they were going to be attacked and raped by them. And he pressed some of my buttons, about our – my – potential to inflict violence on others, and what it is to be a man in a world in which people of my gender inflict pain and suffering on others, and on women in particular.'

'Sounds like he has brought some heavy issues into the counselling and your openness has meant it has not been easy for you.'

'No, I mean, yes, it's not easy, but, well . . .' Graham took a deep breath and connected with his feelings and thoughts. 'I was left wondering just how I might have been, if I had been brought up somewhere like, say, in Northern Ireland. Could I have developed into a "man of violence", whichever side of the so-called religious divide? I like to think not, but I realise that I cannot really be sure, given the fear and the indoctrination that takes place.'

'How does that affect you as a counsellor, Oliver?'

Oliver paused before speaking, 'it kind of undermines me, challenges my sense of the kind of person that I am. I guess I have assumed I am not a violent person, but have I the capacity? Is it something we learn, or is it something we have within us waiting to be unleashed, that for some it is encouraged, whilst for others it is discouraged?'

'So it affects the way you perceive yourself?'

'It left me questioning myself, yes, and realising that I don't know. In a way it perhaps makes me more able to empathise, perhaps, with those who do inflict violence. The difference is that they act on an impulse, and I have learned not to, maybe. I don't know. No, no, it isn't always impulse, there are sadistic bastards who are measured and deliberate. I don't know, but I am aware that working with Graham is bringing me face-to-face with the darker side of humanity, the nastier side, and we touched on it in those terms towards the end of his last session, the third so far.'

'So you are being pushed into listening to details about the nastier side of human expression?'

'And it's very tiring, very draining, and it's like a stain. Wasn't it Shelley who wrote: 'Life, like a dome of many colours, stains the white radiance of eternity'? Or am I misquoting, but it was something like that. I'm sure it wasn't what he meant, but for me it comes to mind because there is something about human life, human expression, that is like a stain, it stains something pure. Like Rogers, I do believe that there is a tendency towards realising potential, and I would say a tendency towards goodness in people. I know that everyone has their beliefs, but it seems to me that life is a journey and it involves growth and goodness in some way, but there are people who seem to want to stain that goodness – I'm tempted to say evil here, for that's what it feels like. And I don't want it to sound religious, I don't see it like that, and yet, at times I am left wondering about it and listening to Graham has sharpened this up for me, brought it into focus.'

'So he's forcing you to confront the problem of good and evil in the world?'

'Yes, well not just out there, inside me as well. And I know that people are shaped and conditioned into ways of thinking, into feelings, into behaviours, and that given the therapeutic conditions then there is an opportunity for people to re-define themselves and in a sense begin to "dis-identify" with aspects of themselves that they wish to reject. And I know all the stuff about contrasting the person that I experience myself as being, and the person I want to be. Oh, I don't know, the words are running away with me.'

'It sounds to me as though something about what Graham is talking about is really disturbing you, I am experiencing you as not having the usual poise that you often bring into our supervision sessions. You seem flustered, disturbed, unsettled.' Jean felt it was important to express what she was perceiving. She knew it was her perception and may not match Oliver's experience, but it felt very present to her as she observed Oliver and listened to the manner of his speech. 'I also had the sense at the start that you introduced Graham in a very matter-of-fact manner, and that's not your usual way.'

'Yes, well, that's Graham, maybe I'm more disturbed than I thought. Maybe it has got to me more than I thought it had, and if so, thank goodness I have some time here to recognise it and work with it.'

'So, feeling disturbed by what Graham is saying, and the question then is around how that is impacting on your ability to offer the therapeutic conditions?'

'I'm not saying much, but my sense is that often Graham is engaging with his own internal world, his memories, thoughts and feelings, and I remember feeling I didn't want to take him away from his relationship with himself by drawing attention to his relationship with me.'

'That's OK, sometimes it is enough to be present and attentive. Clients are good at picking up on whether their counsellor is really listening, you know.'

'Well, it feels right, but I suppose if I am finding it disturbing then I need to be attentive to myself and my own reactions, to be open in my awareness to what I am experiencing, and be able to communicate it when it is appropriate, when it is emerging through the therapeutic relationship.'

'And do you think that is happening?'

'I think so. There was a period in the last session where we both sat in tears.'

'You *both* were in tears, you must have been very affected.'

'I was. Graham talked about a woman they found hanging from a tree, she had hung herself to stop the soldiers finding her. And there was a photo of her I remember seeing in the papers at the time, and it affected me then, and it affected me in the session, and it affects me now as I talk about it.' Oliver's eyes had watered.

'So, yes, you both had feelings to express about that poor woman's death?'

'And in a way I think it moved the therapy on.'

'I'm sure it did. It must have helped Graham to have his own feelings validated, to witness your reaction.'

'We reached a point of there being nothing to say. Maybe if I hadn't had my experience, maybe he might have said more, but there was a kind of meeting, a sort of mutual moment, but I wonder if I blocked him from further exploration, or whether that mutuality was more important and of more therapeutic value. I don't know, and yet I suppose I believe that it was because I think those deep, shared moments caused something to happen, and for both of us.'

'Mhmm, both of you ...' Jean nodded and smiled as she responded, struck herself by the image of two men meeting in such a profound way. She was sure Oliver's reaction would have validated Graham's feelings and maybe helped him to own and be aware of his feelings more, and maybe communicate them more openly.

An important way of thinking about congruence is in terms of what is present as an experience within the person, their awareness of it and their ability to communicate what they are aware of. If a person has accurate awareness of their experiencing, and can communicate it freely without distortion, then congruence is present. But where there is a breakdown in the internal relationship, then incongruence will be present. So, if something is present within the person in terms of their experience but they are unaware of it, then they cannot be congruent, or perhaps that something may be communicated through a tense posture but this is something that the person is oblivious too, then again there has to be a state of incongruence.

Elsewhere I have described this relationship and shown how the flow of experience into awareness and communication can be affected/disrupted by alcohol and therefore manifest incongruence (Bryant-Jefferies, 2001).

'And, you know, what I guess has just suddenly struck me, and I hadn't realised this before, but now it seems somehow so important to acknowledge, but I have met one of the men who found that woman, and I have witnessed his pain, and he has witnessed mine . . .' Oliver closed his eyes. 'It makes the image more personal, and it feels important for me to react as a human-being to that event.'

'So the sharing of your pain has highlighted the importance of reacting in a very human way.'

'There is something about pain, about being able to feel another's hurt, or should I say to be able to feel hurt in the presence of hurt.'

'Feeling hurt within yourself when in the presence of the hurt of another?'

Oliver was looking slightly to the side of Jean. 'It is important for me to feel that hurt, to feel that pain, to be touched, affected. It's the price of love.' Oliver looked up as he spoke those last five words. 'It's the price of love.' His voice had softened as he repeated it.

'Hurt and pain – the price of love?' Jean wasn't questioning what Oliver was saying, but seeking to hear a little more as to what Oliver was meaning.

'Yes. And I'm not really sure what I mean, but I remember some years ago reading a book in which there was this phrase, and it made an impression on me. It must have made a deep impression as I've never forgotten it: The "sharp shears of sorrow must separate the real from the unreal; the lash of pain must awaken the sleepy soul to exquisite life; the wrenching away of the roots of life from the soil of selfish desire must be undergone, and then the man stands free" (Bailey, 1960). It just seems that there is something about love and pain, love and sorrow, that love or compassion is borne out of pain, and in a world with so much pain and sorrow, there is an opportunity for so much more compassion. Maybe that's what pain is for, to unlock compassion, to awaken more human hearts, I don't know. Maybe I'm losing the plot.'

'Now, let me see if I am hearing you. Feeling your client's pain encourages compassion in you, yes? It kind of evokes a compassionate response. This is what happens in therapy, but not just in therapy. And therefore the more people who are affected by the pain of others, the more scope there is for compassion in the world?'

'Something like that, and I think that in the moment when that happens, then the unconditional positive regard that we speak of becomes truly heartfelt, no, I mean . . . What do I mean? It's like, my caring for my client is genuine and there is some kind of heart-to-heart connection – it is like my heart feels their pain and in that moment maybe their heart feels my pain and my compassion and something other, something deeper, something, I guess, spiritual, happens. I'm not sure quite what I mean, but I just have a sense that there is something beyond unconditional positive regard, that whilst I can hold this attitude and these acceptant feelings, there is a sense that I am making it so. But with compassion, there is a spontaneity, there is nothing that I am doing, there is no attitude I am holding, there is simply the presence of compassion and I am convinced that there is a quality of healing that becomes present in those moments that goes beyond the usual therapeutic experience.' Oliver stopped speaking. The words had just flowed from his mouth, and he felt good about what he had said. He hadn't quite put it that way before, but somehow it had come together, and he was aware of awaiting Jean's reaction.

'Like a depth of unconditional positive regard that somehow transcends – that's an interesting contradiction – but it somehow extends beyond something that you are doing as a counsellor.'

'As a person, I think it's bigger than counselling.'

'As a person, OK, so there can be moments when the pain of your client can open you, as a counsellor, as a person, to a moment of compassion, a kind of transcending moment in some way? And I am thinking of Buber's *I-Thou* relationship.'

'I think so. But I think what happened with Graham was that we both realised our pain for the same event, and somehow, in that moment, it was like we dissolved and all that remained was the pain and then the compassion. It was fleeting, but it was there, and then it was gone.'

'A moment of connection and a fleeting moment of compassion.'

'And then it moved on, Graham said something about mass graves and, yes, I made a response that, well, something about his having buried his feelings under the corpses. But I missed something as well, he talked of the smell of death and I didn't pick up on that, and yet he spoke of how haunting it was, at least I think that was what he said.'

'So you think you lost contact with him on that?'

'I think so. It was intense, but that's not an excuse. And in a way what I said was true as well. So many different strands. Later he did experience a shift, differentiating the corpses and the faces of the women from the perpetrators of the atrocities. Or rather differentiating his feelings. That felt important, a definite ''moment of movement'', I think. He talked of feeling damaged and I think realised that he had thought of the experiences he had had as being the cause of the damage, but realised in the session that the perpetrators were the real cause, it was their inhumanity that had damaged him, not the victims however much those images were with him. I think it helped him move his feelings to where they needed to be focused. That seemed like a big step.'

Jean was nodding. 'Perhaps his feelings towards the victims will change, maybe it will let in more compassion for him, and perhaps the images will be less disturbing in some way?'

'Maybe.'

'We've covered a lot of ground, Oliver, and I wonder if there is anything more you feel you need to say about Graham, and how you feel about working with him. Has what we have discussed helped you to be how you need to be when you next see him?'

'I wonder how many Graham's there are in the world, Jean, coping as best they can with memories. I know I worked with a few when I did alcohol counselling at an agency a few years back. Men who drank to forget, or to numb feelings, or because they couldn't adapt to civilian life. And Graham's struggled with that one as well, and he's made a few references to drinking, but nothing has come out to indicate a real problem.'

'But you don't plan to mention it?'

'No, I'd need to be experiencing concern, real concern, to bring it up, and then it would be an expression of my warmth and concern for him, and in a way that would be sensitive to the context. I don't know. Maybe I wouldn't. It's a difficult one. Always a difficult area when you know something that a client may not appreciate. But it's not an issue that Graham is presenting me with.' Oliver smiled, 'I have a lot of respect for Graham, you know. There's something good about him. The way he speaks about his experiences, there's a lot of sensitivity there and he must have had to bury that to deal with the situations he's had to face – hence my comment about his burying his feelings under the corpses. I hope he can come to terms with it all and maybe find an outlet for that sensitivity as he regains more and more awareness of his feelings.'

'You think that is how it will unfold?'

'I think he's on a journey to regain his feelings, regain his sensitivity, and in doing that has a lot of experiences to address. I will offer him the therapeutic conditions, continue to be touched and affected I am sure by the material he brings – what a phrase, "the material he brings". That's real counsellor-speak. Maybe I should say I will be touched and affected by his process of becoming, but I'm not sure that's any better. No, humour aside, this *is* serious business. I will stay with him in his process, and I don't know what else will emerge, but I will be there, and I will be affected, and I hope I can openly be myself as a person, as a man, as a counsellor – and maybe in that order, but that's another discussion. So, yes, I feel prepared to listen to him and share what he brings to the session.'

Points for discussion

- What do you regard as the key purpose of supervision, and do you think that was fulfilled in this session?
- Do you feel everything was addressed that needed to be? If you were Jean, would you have responded differently to Oliver at any time during the supervision session, and if so, why?
- What else might you have brought to supervision had you been Oliver?
- How effective did you feel Jean was as a supervisor? Was her supervision practice congruent with person-centred principles?
- What do you think Oliver would have taken from the supervision session, and how might it effect how he is with Graham in the next session?
- Does the pain and sorrow of the client draw compassion from the heart of the counsellor? If so, how does that relate to person-centred theory?
- Write notes for the session as if you are Oliver.

CHAPTER 14

Counselling session 4: a deeper cathartic release and a more conversational exchange

'I haven't been sleeping too well. I don't know why, I thought that releasing those feelings last week may have made a difference, but I'm not sure that it has.'

'What was different about last week?' Oliver realised he had directed Graham, he needed to get his focus, he was somehow out of step with him and he wasn't sure why.

'Apart from the sleeping, it began OK. No problem the night after I left here, actually I slept well, but it sort of creeps up on you. I just found myself feeling drained, exhausted by it all, and then at night I couldn't settle. In the past it has always been the corpses and the smell that has stayed with me so much. And that's there to a degree, but it's the women I met over there, who I talked about last week, that image is much more vivid now, and I wake up feeling helpless, like I don't know what to do. My heart is pounding, I'm sweating, and I feel, well, it's like being asked to do something but you don't know how to do it. I see faces, pleading with me to help them, and they are images that aren't exactly as I remember it, it's like my mind has got hold of it all and distorted it. And there's nothing I can do. And that leaves me disturbed for the rest of the night. I do sleep, but I don't feel rested. Hence I'm feeling so tired.'

'So the images aren't as you remember them, but certainly drawn from what you witnessed.'

'Mmm. It just leaves me unsettled. In a way, it's not so much the dreams as the effect, that feeling of just not being able to settle back into sleep.'

'So it's the way you are left feeling after you have woken up?'

Graham nodded.

'Can you say a little more about those feelings?'

'I feel sweaty, sort of on edge, just unsettled really. My mind races, I'm thinking of all kinds of things, stupid things usually, but a real mix. Sometimes about work and whether I'll get back to work and stuff like that, then things around the house, or what Angela's doing or the kids, never anything in particular. And that's as well as the memories from the past that are there.'

151

'So it's as though your mind is overactive when you wake up and it's hard to
stop it.'

'I lie there, try to find a comfortable position, I get hot, I get up, walk around the
house, sometimes watch something on TV.'

'It's often good to get out of the bedroom when you can't sleep.'

'Well, I do that. I might read the paper, though I've usually already been through
it. I've tried crosswords, but can't seem to concentrate enough.'

'So there's something about not being able to settle after you've woken up, and
your sense is that the dreams wake you up?'

Graham nodded again.

'And the dreams are about feeling helpless before the women that you remember
from Bosnia?'

Graham nodded again. He was tight-lipped as he felt his mind go back to the past
once more. 'You know, it's crazy, but I remember hearing that the thing they
sent in to the women was lipstick! Can you believe it, but apparently it helped.
Didn't solve anything but psychologically . . . I'd never have thought of that.'

'Sounds like it's the kind of thing that maybe you wished you could have
thought of?'

'I suppose you are right. I didn't know what to do, what to say. There wasn't anything. I'm not trained to deal with a situation like that, none of us were. And we
were men as well, and that didn't help. Fortunately there were women in the
area with the UN as well, and they were brought over, and that made a difference. I couldn't help them, all I could have done would have been to capture or
kill the men that had done it. That's what I'm trained to do. They'd long gone.
I didn't know what to do.'

'Didn't know what to do.' Oliver stayed focused on the feeling that Graham was
expressing. His sense was that this feeling of – well, the word impotence was in
his mind – was the real trauma, the feeling of being faced with such horror and
not knowing what to do.

'I was trained to know what to do, Oliver, trained to know how to act, how to
react, how to deal with pressure situations, how to stay disciplined. Years and
years, I could do all that standing on my head, but there I was, and I can feel
myself standing there now, trees over to the right, the makeshift buildings
ahead of me, barbed wire all around, and it was grey, cloudy, a damp wind in
my face. I can see it, feel it, and I could only look.' He took a short, sharp breath.
'I've seen the films of the concentration camps. This was different. That was
someone else's war, this was mine, but I didn't know what to do, I didn't
know what to do . . .' The tears began to flow as Graham broke down in front
of Oliver. These were not tears like he had cried before, these were deep, aching
tears that came from deep within his being. These were tears that came from
the heart of a man who having discovered long ago that he wasn't able to be
the man that he thought he was, and who had tried to bury the realisation,
a man whose whole identity had been built on knowing how to cope and what
to do, a man who in a moment of human tragedy and horror had found himself wanting.

Oliver got up and went over to Graham, putting his hand on his shoulder, and giving it a gentle but firm squeeze. Graham lifted his hand and gripped hold of Oliver's hand. The moment passed and the tears flowed, tears locked away for ten years or more. 'I didn't know what to do.' As he spoke the words another wave of emotion hit Graham and his eyes streamed once again, hot tears of pain and frustration. He sniffed and swallowed, and released his grip on Oliver's hand. Oliver reached over for the tissues and handed them to Graham. 'Thanks. Oh sweet Jesus . . .', and another wave of feelings rose up through his body and again filled his eyes with tears. He felt hot, he was burning up. He swallowed again as he felt the wave pass. It was like being amongst waves on a beach, waves of emotion, all bottled up and forcing their way out.

Graham took a deep breath. Oliver gripped his shoulder again and squeezed before returning to his chair.

'A bugger, isn't it?' Graham was shaking his head.

Oliver nodded, 'yeah, yes it is.'

'Oooh,' Graham blew the air out of his mouth and took another deep breath, held it and then let that go as well. 'I've been bottling that lot up, haven't I?'

'I think so.'

'It felt like those tears came from a deep place, and from all of me. Look, I'm shaking.' Graham held up his right arm. His hand was trembling, so was his left.

'I think we store emotion all over our bodies.'

'Funny, that's how it felt, I could feel the emotion inside of me, but my whole body was affected, heavy, hot, burning up.'

'Everywhere heavy, hot and burning.'

Graham had picked up the glass and was sipping the water. It felt cool and refreshing and he followed the cool sensation as it passed down his throat and into his stomach. He breathed deeply again and blew the air out. 'I had no idea.'

'No idea?'

'That I had those feelings, well, that I could cry like that.' Graham was rubbing his eyes with a tissue. 'I must look a state. It's OK for you, I've got to walk out there through the waiting room. Is it always like this in counselling?'

'No, not always, but sometimes. You let a lot out just then.'

'I couldn't hold it back, couldn't control it, didn't even try, it just hit me, well, came at me, from inside me, oh words are useless.'

'Bubbled out.'

'Never mind bubbles, like a volcano. Bang, like someone had cut the top off a volcano under pressure and everything just blew.'

'Must have had the top down firmly for a long time.'

'Without realising it.'

'Takes a lot of energy to achieve that.'

'Is that why I've been tired so much?'

'I don't think we understand emotional energy much, but yes, it could be.'

Graham was shaking his head. 'They call that something, don't they, a . . . , what is it, a catha . . . something reaction?'

'Cathartic reaction.'

'Well, more intense than the other sessions.'

'Yes.'

'How much more?'

'I don't know.'

'It's like cleaning out a wound, isn't it, getting all the pus out.'

'Something like that.'

'And it has to be cleaned right out, doesn't it?'

Oliver nodded, 'yes.'

'So there may be some more surprises?'

'Maybe.'

Graham lifted up his right arm, the trembling had stopped. 'That's something, anyway.'

'How are you now?'

'Yeah, feeling kind of numb, I guess. A bit like the calm that follows a storm. I can feel my heart beating, I bet my pulse is up.'

'It's amazing how we can lock feelings and emotions away, quite unaware that they are there. But now you feel calmer, but aware of your heart beating away.'

'I don't know what to say now. I think I just need to sit here for a bit and, well, just be.' He picked up the glass and finished the water.

'Can I get you some more?'

'Please, thanks.' Oliver took the glass and headed out to refill it. He took his time, allowing Graham to have time to just be with his thoughts and feelings without any sense of pressure to say something that might be there when he was in the room.

He came back in and handed Graham the glass.

'So, no rush, no need to do anything, 20 minutes left, up to you.'

Graham put the glass down and leant back into the chair. 'I'm not sure I feel like saying anything. But it's good to just sit.'

'OK, sure. Do you want me to stay, or leave you to sit?'

'Stay, I'm sure I'll want to say something.'

'Sure, take your time.' Oliver sat back himself and consciously took his attention away from Graham, not wanting his observing of him to become an intrusion.

Graham felt calm, he really did feel calm. He thought back over the past three weeks. He'd only come along four times and it had been like stepping on to some crazy roller-coaster. Now it felt as though there was some respite. Maybe it was stopping and he could get off. No such luck, he thought, it's probably slowly and gently ascending before the next accelerated plunge. The image drifted aside. He was thinking of his wife, of Angela. They'd had problems for a while now, though nothing too serious, but it hadn't been easy, and he guessed that the truth was that he hadn't been easy. He wanted to be different. Maybe he needed to talk to her now, not go into detail, but tell her something about the counselling. She'd asked after each session but he hadn't said much. Maybe he needed to say something about it though he wondered if it would make him upset and how that would be.

'Do you think that I ought to talk to Angela about these counselling sessions?'

'Is that what you feel you'd like to do?'

'Well, I wonder. She does ask but, well, I haven't said much. Just wonder if it might help me, us, if I did.'

'She might appreciate it.'

'I might end up in tears.'

'You might.'

'Mmm. Not sure how she'd react.'

'Not sure how she'd react to you expressing feelings?'

'She'd find it strange.'

'Mhmm.'

'I suppose it has been strange for me too.'

'Uh-hu.'

'You're not going to tell me, are you?'

Oliver shook his head. 'Nope.'

'You don't give advice, do you?'

'Not the way I work. I want people to find their own answers, discover their own resources to deal with situations that have arisen in their lives.'

'Couldn't run an army like that. It would be anarchy.'

They lapsed back into silence. For Oliver this was still therapy. So the usual, in-depth therapeutic encounter had passed by for the session, but it was still about two people in a relationship, and for Oliver it was important that whilst the conversation may become lighter, he would remain aware of the therapeutic aspect to their exchange of words.

Graham shook his head. 'And you're paid for this!'

'Sometimes it is helpful to slow things down, have time like this. Yes, I am paid for it. I'm a skilled professional.' Oliver couldn't resist the comment and the smile that he could feel breaking out on his face.

'Yes, you are that. But you've shown me more than just being a counsellor. You cried with me.' The tears were back in Graham's eyes, as they were in Oliver's.

'I know.'

'I won't forget that.'

'Neither will I.'

They maintained eye contact. 'Time I headed off. Thanks, Oliver. I don't understand this therapy stuff, but I guess you don't need to for it to work.'

'No, you don't need to. But there are plenty of books on it.'

'I think I'm learning more as a client.'

'We're both learning, then.'

Graham put out his hand, Oliver took it, the grip was firm. Two men conveying mutual respect. 'You take care and I hope you have a better week.'

'I think I will. I think last week started what happened this week.'

Graham walked out of the surgery to his car and headed straight home. He didn't think about spending time alone. He wanted to go home. He spent that evening talking to Angela. He didn't say everything, but said a little about the counselling and how it seemed to be affecting him. He didn't give her the details of his military experiences, no, he'd never burden her with those. His army relationships were something else. But he did show emotion and it did bring them closer. That night they made love in a way that they hadn't done in years.

Oliver had watched him walk across the car park to his car, a purposeful stride, clearly he was heading off somewhere with great deliberation. What a session, he thought to himself. And was the last ten minutes or so therapy? It felt therapeutic. He was concerned with getting an appropriate balance of personal and professional. You couldn't be all one or all the other, you needed a blend of both, though he felt strongly that probably the most effective counsellors were those who strayed more towards the personal than the professional end of the spectrum. Or was that just his prejudice because it was how he liked to work?

Points for discussion

- Personal or professional – what balance do you think is most appropriate, and what factors govern this?
- How was unconditional positive regard conveyed in this session, and to what effect?
- What were the key moments and how did Oliver contribute to them during this session?
- How were you feeling when Graham experienced his cathartic reaction? Reflect on why those particular feelings were present for you.
- When the dialogue becomes conversational is it acceptable in a therapeutic context? List the pros and cons. When might it be acceptable, and when not?
- Clearly a relationship is developing between client and counsellor. How would you describe that relationship as an observer, and using your own words?
- Write notes for this session.

CHAPTER 15

Counselling session 5: an act of unlawful killing? And alcohol use is addressed

'Better week?' Oliver could see a marked contrast in Graham's facial expression.

'Yes.' He described his conversation with Angela and the result.

'So, how do you want to use our time today, and we probably need to talk about how many more sessions you want, or feel you need.'

'Sure. I know there's a limit, and I want to try and tie it in with my thinking of going back to work. I spoke to Dr Cross last week and he feels, and I feel, that I need to begin to work towards it. I know I haven't dealt with everything, but I need to be pragmatic as well. I do need to go back to work, I can't wait until I have been through everything in therapy – that's if I need to do that.'

'Sure, I can appreciate that.'

'But if I do go back I'm not sure whether I can still see you, at least to begin with.'

'I do have early evening appointments here, but the latest I start is 6 pm.'

They discussed the options and Graham agreed to check it out with his employer. He thought they'd be agreeable, they appeared very supportive and had been pleased with his work since he had joined the company.

Graham was, however, feeling anxious. He knew that he had given an impression to Oliver that wasn't strictly true and he wasn't sure whether he wanted to disclose another event from his past, one that he had not been very proud of, but which had happened, and had in reality proved to himself that he was capable of premeditated violence although he'd rather think of it as having been a reaction to circumstances. But he really valued his ability to talk with Oliver and did not want to in some way affect Oliver's perception of him. The fact that Oliver had listened and accepted him, and what he had to say, was important, very important. But how would he react? What would happen? He wasn't sure, he wasn't convinced he wanted to say anything and so he kept quiet, at least for now. But because this was in the forefront of his thinking he wasn't really sure what else to say.

'I'm not sure what to talk about this week.'

'So, things to choose from, or nothing feeling very pressing?'

'Nothing feeling very pressing.' He felt uncomfortable saying it.

'So, all seems OK just at the moment, a better week, talking things through with Angela, and thinking about getting back to work before too long.'

Graham nodded. 'Yes.'

Graham is clearly experiencing the anxiety that arises from being incongruent. With Oliver offering the core conditions then the likelihood is that there will be therapeutic movement if the facilitative climate enables Graham to make visible the source of his incongruence.

The dialogue felt somehow stiff to Oliver, but he accepted it and felt sure that if there was a reason for this then when Graham was ready he would say something. Oliver just had a sense that something wasn't quite right. He knew from experience that his own congruence was likely to enhance a client's sense of their own incongruence, sometimes increasing their anxiety until they felt impelled to voice whatever it was that was troubling them, or if it was something they were unaware of, it could seemingly draw it to the surface.

Oliver spoke as he felt. 'Great. I am just aware of how much you have discussed these past few weeks and whilst I know it can only represent a small part of your experience, it has felt to me as though you have talked about some very significant events and connected with profound feelings associated with them. Takes a lot of courage, Graham, and I respect that in you.'

Whilst it was good to hear, Graham was also feeling more uncomfortable. 'Thanks. I don't feel I had much choice once I started. The feelings just erupted, as it were. But, yes, I guess it does take courage, but maybe if I'd known exactly what I was letting myself in for, and then still came, then maybe that would have been courage.'

'You think you might not have come had you known?'

'Don't know. Not an easy question to answer. I hope I would have come, but I can't be sure, not the way I was thinking then, but maybe I would have done, if only to keep the doctor happy!'

'Some people do attend more to please the doctor than because they want to. Not everyone is at ease with coming, and in fact most people are definitely not at ease – that's one of the reasons why they need to come in the first place.' Oliver was aware that they were talking about matters that were keeping the focus away from what was happening for Graham now in the room.

'I wasn't comfortable, I have to say, but I've dealt with people in all kinds of settings and situations, so I felt sure I could deal with this.'

'Feel more comfortable now?'

Graham did in one way, at least he felt comfortable with Oliver as a person, but he felt distinctly uncomfortable in himself. 'Yes.'

'Good.'

They lapsed into silence. Oliver felt absolutely sure there was something happening for Graham, but he wanted to give him every opportunity to find within himself the strength to voice it, if it was the case and he wasn't sitting with a fantasy in his head. But it felt different. The way the session was going, particularly after such a good week, and the ease with which they had been talking at the end of the last session, something was not right.

Graham's heart was pounding a little more strongly and his palms felt a little more sweaty than usual. He had been looking down at the floor, but now he looked up, searchingly. How would Oliver respond?

Oliver saw the look and returned the eye contact. Something was happening, he knew it, and he needed to help Graham voice it. He decided to speak softly and enquire. 'What's eating you, Graham?'

Graham looked away. He shook his head.

'That bad, huh?'

Graham nodded.

'Worse than what you've already told me?'

He nodded.

'I'd really like to hear what it is. If I can help, you know I'll do what I can.'

Graham took a deep breath. Shit, he thought. He had to say it, the thought of that rock in his path, obstructing his way, it was like every time he tried to clear it, there was another one, and another, and they seemed to get bigger.

'It's something I'm not proud of, and it makes me feel very ashamed.'

Oliver nodded. 'OK.' His lips felt tight, and he felt he was frowning a little. He wanted to look open and encouraging of Graham to trust him. 'Not something you're going to find easy to tell me, yeah?'

Graham nodded.

'Take your time, no rush.'

Graham sat in silence for a few moments. 'The Gulf, The Gulf War. I'd shot people before, but always in a battle, always in an exchange of fire, always to achieve an objective and to protect the unit. That's how we were trained.'

'Mhmm, trained to shoot in an exchange of fire and in combat situations, yeah?'

'Well, that was how it should have been, and usually was. Yes, that rule was broken a few times in Northern Ireland, but we could justify that, we had intelligence, we were taking out bombers, crazed people who wanted nothing other than to kill and maim. We were justified. It was a dirty war. We were justified, we did what we had to do. One dead bomber meant a lot of innocent people might live, yes?'

Oliver nodded, aware that this was a preamble and he didn't want to get in the way of what Graham was leading up to.

'Justified, one death meant many others might live.' He spoke in a tone of voice to convey his acceptance of what Graham was saying.

Graham was looking down as he spoke. 'Well, it got a bit different in the Gulf. We were fighting, if fighting is the right word, the Iraqis were so out-gunned, so out-trained it was ridiculous. We were going in behind the tanks, and it was hot and dusty and there was smoke from the oilfields up in flames, a real mess. The Iraqis were retreating. We'd taken out tank after tank. No survivors, not in a tank battle. You're hit, you're dead, they didn't have the armour. We were just picking them off. We came across this place where some Iraqi troops had dug in, most had fled or were dead, two of them were left alive, just young lads,

fear in their faces. Couldn't have been more than 17 or 18. They had their arms up as we approached them. We were close, shouting at them to keep their arms up. One of them must have panicked, started firing, hit Jimmy, took it in the throat, hadn't been aimed, just unlucky, died before he hit the ground, took out his windpipe. The other Iraqi still had his hands up and was shouting, the guy who had fired was now dead, someone had taken him out with a bullet to the head. The one that was left had scrambled out, still with his hands up, desperate for us not to shoot. Jimmy was dead, behind us. The Iraqi wasn't going to fire, he was no threat to us.' Graham was back re-living the scene, walking up to the young Iraqi, flanked by his comrades in arms. He was shaking his head. 'He shouldn't have shot Jimmy. He shouldn't have fired the gun, there was no need, we were taking prisoners, they'd have been OK, they were kids.'
'What happened, Graham?'
Graham was still re-living the scene, it was as though it was being lived out again. He could see his face, the utter terror in his eyes. He wasn't very big, dwarfed against the handful of men in uniform who surrounded him.
'I can hear myself say, "You fucking bastard, you didn't have to kill him." I shot him in the leg, and he fell in agony, and I smashed his face with the rifle butt, again and again. I lost it, big time. I killed him. I don't imagine I was the only one to do it, but I killed him. I didn't need to kill. I really didn't need to do it, but I did.' Graham looked up. 'So you see, I know I can kill in cold blood, not out of threat, not to protect, not to return fire, but needlessly. I can do that. Anywhere else, it would have been murder. We buried them under the sand and moved on. Someone, somewhere, lost a son that day because I lost control. I have to live with that. I can make excuses. But there aren't any, not really.'
Oliver nodded slightly, as Graham lifted his head. 'Maybe it was for Geordie, all those years before, or maybe it was for Jimmy, or for the untold thousands of dead in Bosnia, or the women in the rape camp, or for the others who died in Northern Ireland, I don't know, I just don't know. But I guess he was the wrong person, in the wrong place, at the wrong time. Who he was, I don't know and can never know. I thought I could bury him beneath the sand and walk away. I walked, but he stayed with me.' He took a deep breath. 'That's how it is. I think of him sometimes, and I think about what I know I'm capable of doing. More than anything else it's that which makes me drink. And it may seem crazy to hear someone in the army talking of drinking to try and forget that he killed someone, but that's the reality. And it's been harder these past 18 months, my son is now the age of that Iraqi soldier, and he reminds me on the bad days of the young life I took because I couldn't control my anger.'
'I don't know what to say, Graham, but I can accept that you lost it because of all that had happened before. And, yes, I can only guess at what it has been like, is like, living with that knowledge.'
'Can't blame anyone else. I did it, and now I can't forget it, and I drink to forget.'
'And it doesn't help.'
Graham shook his head. 'Maybe sometimes, helps me sleep, but usually it doesn't. This I haven't told Angela, and I know I never will. I have to live with it, with the knowing of what I'm capable of. You see, I think of the women's faces in the

rape camp, and somewhere there's an Iraqi mother, and she has a face too, but I can't see it. I can't see it, but it's there.'

'You can't see her face, but you know it's there, that she's out there. It really did affect you, has affected you, and maybe in its own way more than anything else.'

'Everything else was what others had done. But this was me. Yeah, this was me.'

Oliver stayed silent. Graham's words, "this was me", seemed to hang in the air.

'I need help on this one, Oliver, alcohol's not the answer. I know it, but it's getting out of control. I have to deal with it. If I can't, well, it's like cancer inside me, as you said at the start, "what's eating you". That's how it feels. When you said those words I knew I had to tell you. I didn't want to. I feel ashamed. As I've said, I cannot justify my actions. But I pay the price. I pay the price.'

'A heavy price.'

'I guess some would say that I have to live with it, and others that it was nothing, casualty of war, but we're all casualties of war, whatever side, we are all diminished by it, we are all affected.'

'No tears?'

'I've cried over many years, usually on the way to the bottom of a bottle. I don't think there are any left for this one. I just carry the guilt, and the knowing. I have to address the drinking, Oliver, can you help me with that?'

'Yes, do you want to spend time looking at that?'

Oliver moves into more of an alcohol-counselling mode. He is responding to a direct request from Graham for specific help. The relationship has been established. There is a strong rapport between them. Oliver has knowledge of alcohol work and can appreciate the need for Graham to start to try and address the issue. He knows he may be able to offer advice. He has checked whether Graham wants to spend time on his drinking.

Graham nodded. 'I hope by talking today I may ease something. It feels like over these weeks I've been peeling off layers, but I know that this is the last layer, this is the one that lies at the core of it all. I thought, hoped, I could cope without going near it, but, well, here I am, and now you know.'

'Yes, it can be like layers of an onion.'

'So how do I stop drinking on it?'

'What's the pattern?'

'Most nights, a few whiskies late in the evening, and a few more if I wake up in the night.'

'How long does it take you to get through a bottle?'

'Couple a week.'

'Litre bottle or 70 centilitres?'

'The latter, 70 centilitres.'

'Specialist scotch or run of the mill?'

'Run of the mill. Couldn't afford the fancy stuff! I drink to forget, not for the taste.'

'Sixty units a week, not enough to be chemically dependent, but enough to be harmful and to upset sleep patterns.'

'I thought it helped me sleep?'

'Yes, and no. Helps you sleep by relaxing you, alcohol is a suppressant, but it's knock-out sleep, not natural sleep. Tends to upset the natural rhythm, makes it harder to then sleep without alcohol.'

'Yeah, that's true. So, what do I do?'

'I'm coming out of my usual counselling role, here, because I know that there are ideas that can be helpful that people might not otherwise think of. At the same time, I want to encourage you to think about what you feel you could do to change the pattern that has got established.'

'Well, I have to drink less, I have to cut back, maybe just try and pour out smaller amounts.'

'Mhmm, OK.'

'Try and make a bottle last longer, give myself a quota.'

'That can be good, lines on the bottle, that kind of thing.'

'Mhmm.'

'Diluting it would reduce the harmful effect of drinking it.'

'How do you mean?'

'The warm feeling, the burning in your throat, it's actually inflaming the lining. The more you dilute it, the lower the risk of harm.'

'I could try, but water doesn't seem very appealing.'

'Use iced water, or maybe mix it with something else non-alcoholic.'

'OK.'

'And keep a diary. Here, I have some. Used to work for an alcohol-counselling agency and always carry some with me if the topic comes up. I leave it up to you how you want to fill it in.'

'I feel like I've got some ideas to try, Oliver, thanks for all of this. You told me you didn't give advice!'

'I don't but if I know something that might be helpful, then I'm not going to keep it to myself. I don't want you to think that you have to do anything I've said, I'm not setting homework, it's up to you, think about what feels right, what feels possible, and give it a go, and we can make sense of it next week.'

'OK, thanks, I'll do that.'

'Bring it down slowly.'

'Sure, OK.'

'I know we have moved away from what you shared earlier, and I do want to say that I respect you for telling me. I don't hold it against you. I can hear how you feel about it. I hope it has helped talking about it.'

Graham nodded and got up. 'Yes, I think so. But we'll have to see what the week brings.'

'Sure.'

The session moved on to a brief discussion about where Graham felt he was in relation to returning to work. He left the session early as it gave him a little more time to pick up his daughter from school that day.

Points for discussion

- Graham has disclosed an act of unlawful killing. Would you breach confidentiality? If so, why? If not, why? If unsure, discuss in supervision or with colleagues.
- Are you still feeling the same about Graham? Would you have responded differently to the way Oliver responded?
- How do you feel the therapeutic conditions were established in the session? Find evidence for congruence, empathy and unconditional positive regard being communicated by the counsellor, and being received by the client.
- Was Oliver right to change his way of working when the topic of alcohol use came up? How would you have handled this?
- Write notes for this session.

CHAPTER 16

Counselling session 6: alcohol use and controlling intrusive memories

Graham had felt a little easier during the week, though memories and images remained very present for him. He had the drinking diary with him and he was also keen to work out with Oliver what else he could be offered by way of counselling to help him continue to get himself together.

'So, where do you want to start? And I'm aware that we also need to think ahead of this session as well.' Oliver wanted to leave it open but also ensure that factors that needed to be discussed were flagged up from the start.

'I've been thinking about that and the past week I have been more active around the house, just feeling a little more able to get on with things, and that has felt good. But I feel tired still, and sleep isn't good. I've cut back a bit on the drinking but I think you were right, it hasn't helped my sleeping. I'm still keen to get back to work and I'm aiming for a couple of week's time. I hope that's not too ambitious, but I've been in touch with my boss – he's from a military background as well, and has been really good. I think he's experienced something similar to me, so that must have helped. Anyway, I do want to continue. I'm sure there is more I need to talk about and I want to get the drinking under control, and my sleeping right, and just be normal, I guess.'

'Mhmm, so quite a number of areas to focus on. Where do you want to start?'

'Well, it would be good to know how many more sessions with you.'

'OK, well, I guess that depends on what happens when you go back to work. Did you find out if you can get time off to come?'

'Yes, that's OK, if we can go for that late afternoon/early evening appointment.'

'That's OK, I can offer that to you. And I wonder about another six sessions, that will take you through the point when you return to work, and a little beyond. We don't have to keep it weekly – if you wanted to you could spread the sessions out towards the end. Some people prefer this, others not, we can discuss that over the next couple of sessions, maybe.'

'And what if I did feel I wanted more?'

'Not sure on that. I'd need to discuss the situation with Dr Cross. And you might want to as well. If you do still want counselling and we can't offer it to you –

there being a limit to the number of sessions we can offer, then you might want to look for a private counsellor, and we can give you a list of people.'

Counsellors in GP surgeries cannot refer clients to themselves to be seen privately. Good practice is to provide a list of known, local counsellors, leaving the client to choose. But the issue remains as to why counselling is so often time-limited, even when need exceeds what is on offer. It is one of the few areas where treatment is clearly rationed on the basis of cost. Counsellors working in this setting need to have dealt with their own attitudes towards time-limited working.

'No, I think I'd rather use the time I have with you and then see how I get on.'

'Sure, that's fine. Some people choose to do that, and may at some future point come back for a few sessions if they feel they need to check something out, or if something else has come up, but that would mean Dr Cross referring you back to me.'

'OK.' Graham paused. 'I suppose the next thing is what to focus on.'

'Mhmm, what do you want to focus on?'

'I want to talk about this.' He held up the drinking diary sheet. 'Maybe that's the place to start, and see how it goes from there.'

The next 15 minutes were spent reviewing Graham's drinking pattern and coming up with further ideas as to how he might reduce a little more. He had cut back, he was taking longer to get through a bottle, but was still above the government's recommended safe drinking limit of three to four units a day for men.[3]

'I know my sleep isn't too good, and I'm still tired, but I do feel as though I have a little more energy, at least, I am doing more. And I'm not dwelling on the past so much, although I still am as well.'

'Sure, so in spite of the sleep problems and the tiredness you have more energy to do things, and that's different?'

'It is. I mean, yes, I still think about the past. Well, it's more that the thoughts impose themselves on me.'

'Kind of intrude into your head, as it were?'

'Something like that. I can be doing something, or nothing, thinking about something, or nothing, and then I'm back in the past.'

'Anything in particular?'

'Faces, people. Sometimes people I've known, who were killed or I've lost touch with. Incidents that happened. It still all feels very real.'

'Vivid, huh?'

'Very much so. And the things I've talked about, I think of them as well, and they are still clear, and I do get anxious, particularly at night, not so much in the

---

[3] For a more detailed overview of working with clients on alcohol issues, *see* Bryant-Jefferies (2001; 2003c).

day. I feel more settled in the day, but I'm still waking up at night and then not being able to settle back to sleep. As I've said, I'm making myself not drink alcohol now if I wake up in the night. I'm reading magazines which I'm making sure I have a good supply of, and drinking tea, or fruit juice, and yes, decaffeinated tea.'

'It will pass, the difficulty in sleeping, but clearly the memory circuits are still firing up regularly at night.'

'Yes. And that's the problem. How do I stop that happening?'

'Something to stop you thinking about the past, or at least, those aspects of the past that leave you unsettled.'

Graham thought for a moment. 'I can't use alcohol to switch it off, but I do need a switch.'

'Mhmm, something to switch off the thoughts that you don't want to have.'

'They go round in my head, like they're stuck there. If I could in some way get them out, bit like talking about them here, but it needs something more, I can't call you in the middle of the night!'

'Er, no, I do keep that boundary, but to be serious what I am hearing is your sense that if you could do something with those thoughts at the time, then maybe it might ease things.'

'Well I can't talk to myself. So I don't know. How do people stop themselves thinking things that they don't want to think?'

'I guess by either thinking about something else, or expressing the feelings they have so that they feel more in control of them.'

'It's the control I want. If I could feel in control, that would help.'

'OK, so what would feel like being in control?'

'Choosing when to think them, and when not to.'

'Mhmm, being able to choose to switch them on and off.'

'But that's what I can't do, so I need something else and maybe that will come along later.'

'Mhmm, OK, so forget about controlling the on and off, it's about controlling them when they are present.'

Graham pondered. 'I like the idea about thinking about something else, but that's back to switching them off, and whilst I read the magazines and maybe watch TV, the memories can intrude or re-surface.'

Oliver nodded. He wanted to avoid telling Graham specifically what to do, but he had an idea in his mind. He stayed with his empathy. 'So, putting switching them off aside, the thoughts are there, the memories are in your head, you are sitting experiencing them, what can you do?'

'I could write them down.'

Oliver restrained a smile, that was what he was hoping Graham would say.

'That sounds good, so write them down, get them out on to paper. See what happens.'

'At least I'd be doing something and feeling in control of what I was doing.'

'That's right. So writing them down, expressing them, getting them out of your head and on to paper, yes?'

Graham nodded. 'I can see myself doing that.'

'That seems important, it's something you can imagine yourself doing.'

'Yes, I can. I have written a bit in the past – used to write poetry at one point, not sure where it came from, nothing fantastic of course. But, yes, maybe, maybe . . .' Graham was imaging himself writing what he was thinking. 'How much detail?'

'How much would you want?'

'I think I'd need to write everything, and maybe that would make me more tired as well.'

'Maybe.' Oliver maintained his focus, allowing Graham to make his own suggestions, simply letting him know that he had heard and giving him time to develop his idea.

'OK, I'll give it a go. But I'm going to type it, not handwrite it. I'm more used to using a keyboard these days.'

'As you wish, whatever feels right for you.'

'Memoirs!'

'You've been through a lot, who knows . . .'

'Who'd read it?'

'Whoever would want to know what it is like to be in the kind of situations that you have experienced.'

'No, I need to write it for me. It'd be a bonus if anything else came of it, but no, keep my feet on the ground here.'

'Mhmm, do it in a way that feels right for you, that helps you to control and express the memories.'

Graham was nodding to himself. Yes, it did make sense, he would give it a go. He could see how it would give him some control, get the thoughts out of his head, and make him tired, all at the same time.

'It can't be that simple, can it?'

'You doubt it?'

'Well, it just seems so obvious once you think about it.'

'The trick is the "once you think about it", remember, it's your idea, you thought about it.'

'OK, I'll give it a go.' Graham lapsed into silence. He didn't feel he needed to say any more about that, and they'd looked at the drinking. He was still aware of thoughts and feelings linked to the previous week's session.

'You know, I've talked a lot and, well, really felt some emotion here with you.'

Oliver nodded but did not interrupt.

'It does make me wonder, you know, well, what you think about it all.'

'You wonder what I think about, what, everything, or some things in particular?'

'Well, you said you hadn't been in the military, and it is a different world, it really is. That's why it can be so fucking difficult when you get out. It's a kind of, well, it is, it's a kind of institution, you get used to it. Everything is clear. You have a clear role, clear tasks. You work hard, you play hard. You do a good job and the army looks after you. You make good mates.' He paused. Yeah, he thought to himself, fucking good mates. 'And you'd die for each other. But a lot of people don't understand it, don't want to understand it. For me it's a way of life.'

Oliver noted the present tense, and realised that for Graham he still very much lived through a sort of military sense of self. 'So, people don't understand but for you that way of life is your way of life.'

'I like clarity. I like, well, like we just discussed. I've got something to go and do to cope with my thoughts, I like that. It's clear.'

'Mhmm, and it's important for you to have that clarity.'

'It is. It's like the military mind: sees a problem, breaks it down, comes up with solutions and implements them.'

'That's how you like to function, yes?'

'And yet, this counselling, and don't get me wrong, it's clearly making a difference, but so much of what has happened here has been, well, I don't know what's been going on. I talk, you listen, you say a few things, and I'm in tears.' Graham was shaking his head. 'I really don't grasp it.'

'So the fact that we haven't sat down and broken the problem down, formulated strategies and implemented them leaves you, what . . . ?'

'Unclear, I guess, as to what it's all about.'

'All a bit of a mystery, huh?' Oliver smiled, and knew that maybe he should be a little more serious, but the relationship felt as though it had developed enough to contain a bit of humour.

'Mystery to me, but it works, it helps. It's like what I said about writing things down, is it that simple? Sit down, talk about stuff, get all upset and move on. Is it that simple?' Graham really was perplexed by it all, and yet he had to admit that there was something attractive, no, compelling about coming and talking in the way he did, with Oliver. Yes, he'd had his doubts at the start, but now he, well, the thought in his mind was that he had perhaps become a convert, though he wasn't quite sure what to.

'You might want to read some books about it. There are lots of approaches to counselling, I base my practice on "the person-centred approach".' Oliver said a little about Carl Rogers, but without getting into too much detail and then brought the focus back. 'It isn't simple. It's actually quite disciplined, and I use that word deliberately mindful that it will have a meaning for you too.'

'Yes, that's interesting, I can see what you mean. You don't just say anything, do you, it's quite deliberate, quite measured.'

'What I say flows from my experience of what I feel you are saying or communicating, and what I am experiencing in myself in response to what you are saying.'

Graham nodded. Oliver was aware that the notion of therapeutic exchange was perhaps now being stretched somewhat in this session, but he also knew from experience that there often was a point in the counselling process when a client could become interested in what it was all about, and it felt right to address that when the interest was present and alive to the client.

'So, you don't just say anything?'

'No. It has to be in response to you, or if it comes from me it has to feel as though it is related to what is happening here and now, in the room, in the therapeutic relationship.'

'This may not be what we should be talking about, but I'm interested, I really am. So you are telling me that being a counsellor is a very disciplined profession, let's say?'

'I can only speak for myself and my own experience. The way that I work requires me to be disciplined, and that means I have to know myself well enough to be able to maintain that disciplined approach with my clients. At the same time, discipline does not mean closed, I have to be open as well; fluid, responsive, yes?'

'Yes. Mmm. You've given me something to think about. Fascinating. And it's making a difference for me.'

'I'm pleased to hear it. But different people work at different paces. It can be a short or long process, and either can be torturous, of course.'

'OK. Thanks for that.' Graham had noticed the time. 'Is that the time, almost time to end.'

'So, I hope that has helped throw a bit of light on what this strange phenomenon called counselling is all about.'

'It's beginning to seem not so strange.' Graham, stood up. 'Thanks, I'll see you next week.'

Graham left and Oliver returned to his seat wondering if Graham was taking his own first step to becoming a counsellor himself. He knew how often clients took it up. Maybe that path was ahead for Graham. In a way, he silently hoped that he would take the path, and then wondered if he had talked at too much length about counselling because of this although at the time he hadn't really thought about it quite like that. He knew he had to watch that, else the sessions could end up as theoretical discussions, and, well, if that was what Graham needed at the moment as part of his process, was it really that wrong to accept that?

'Well', he heard himself saying out loud, 'if he can come through sorting out the issues from his life so far, maybe he'll make a good counsellor'. And particularly to people affected by warfare, he then thought to himself, if he could keep his empathy focused on the client's world and not drift into his own past – always an issue when people counsel others whose experiences are so close to their own.

Oliver took a deep breath. Would the writing help? He wasn't sure, but it was Graham's idea and maybe it would be helpful for him. If he could break the cycle of thoughts and memory intrusions. Yes, he had witnessed disturbing events and in some ways it was right not to forget them, but if they could be remembered in a way that was controlled, and what they provided could be used to enhance the qualities of the person in some way, that had to be for the good.

Points for discussion

- What is your reaction having read Graham's counselling sessions with Oliver? Clarify for yourself why you have this particular reaction.
- Evaluate Oliver's empathic responding during this session.
- Was it appropriate for the session to include a discussion about counselling?

- Do you think Graham might make a good counsellor, if so why, if not, why, and list the 'fors' and 'againsts'.
- What stands out for you from Graham's counselling sessions with Oliver? What were the key moments?
- Write notes for this session.

Reflections on the process

Oliver's reflections – 'I feel very much in a therapeutic relationship with Graham. We seem to have gelled in some way; there is an ease in our interactions. It had felt that it had been developing before the fifth session, and that session then felt a little more stuck because Graham was unsure whether to communicate the incident in the Gulf. But I think that also helped to clear away an obstacle and it feels like we have moved on.

'Maybe the rest of the sessions will be focused on the changes he is making now, as well as handling going back to work. But I am also aware that he is intent on writing down his thoughts, feelings and memories, and this may provide material for future sessions. How the balance will be between the different areas of his life, I do not know. And that feels good. I want it to be open and expressive. I want to offer a therapeutic environment in which Graham can bring himself and whatever is present for him.

'I want to add something about discipline. Person-centred practice *is* a discipline. It's often seen by some as being woolly, or vague, and worse still an approach that sanctions "anything goes" because a counsellor is supposedly being congruent – the "I feel, therefore I express" or "I think therefore I voice" school of pseudo person-centredness. The person- or client-centred counsellor must be self-aware and self-disciplined, and yet fluid and open. And that is the challenge, and by rising to this challenge we offer opportunity to our clients, opportunity for them to flourish as persons, and in a way that is less affected by "conditions of worth" and the "external loci of evaluation" that can so undermine an individual's potential and personhood.

'We have touched on some challenging areas of human experience, life and death, does it get more challenging than that? I have been extended by it, and I welcome that. The intensity and nature of the issues Graham brought to me, and will bring to me, I am sure, in the next few sessions, have forced me to look at myself, my prejudices, my feelings.

'The key moments for me may be the same as those for Graham, but they may not be. And I know immediately what stands out. Crying with him as we both recalled the woman in Bosnia hanging from the tree. Somehow, my being affected by that photo all those years before suddenly took on a fresh meaning as I realised Graham had been there and had actually seen her hanging there. My experience meant that I could genuinely react to him in the way that I did. I felt good about that reaction. It felt genuinely human, and there was something "man-to-man" about that moment which for me went beyond what we generally think of as being a "man-to-man" moment.

'So, I am sure I will never forget these sessions, and I will be changed as a result, even though I may not immediately know what all those changes are. And I still marvel at the connectedness of life, how paths cross or coincide, how events and memories ripple through time to suddenly emerge with added meaning and purpose in the future. I don't believe in chance.'

Graham's reflections – 'Well, I certainly wasn't too enthusiastic at the start. Counselling was for people who couldn't cope, couldn't handle themselves or life. Load of wishy-washy nonsense. Men like me don't cry, you get on with it, you support the people around you. You do what has to be done. You have to be mentally tough. It's trained into you. Now, well, now I'm thinking a bit differently. And I still can't really make sense of it, but the evidence is in front of me, well, actually it's inside of me. I feel different. It's not that I haven't stopped thinking about the past, and being affected by it, but it's becoming different and I hope that continues. But why sitting down and talking and getting all emotional has made that happen, well it's still a mystery, and I really must read some of the books by Rogers. Seems to me he's got something.

'It's hard to know what to say. Still got a few sessions to go, not sure what we'll talk about, but I'm sure I'll think of something. I still have a lot to sort out, but knowing I have a few more sessions will keep me focused I'm sure.

'I wonder what Oliver is writing about the work he has done with me. I say "work" because I'm sure that's what it must feel like to him, it certainly has to me. Exhausting! But he told me at the start he has someone called a "supervisor" to talk things through with. Bloody good idea, could have done with that myself in the past. I'm sure a lot of problems in life could be resolved if those responsible for people had someone to discuss things with and maybe unload their own frustrations on. But without getting emotional. No, the military focus must be free of emotion.

'I know at the start it felt a bit irritating hearing Oliver telling me what I'd just said, didn't feel right. Maybe he should have warned me. Could have put me off. But then it sort of became OK, quite helpful really. Often he wasn't saying exactly what I'd said, and it made me think, what did I mean, what was I feeling. Yes, so what seemed unhelpful turned out to be, well, helpful. But I don't think he really understood me, not really. You have to have been in combat to know what it is like. He tried, and I suppose I tried to help him understand as well. Maybe if he'd had a military background . . . I don't know. It would have been different.

'For me the most important moment was, well, the moment when I realised that it wasn't the victims that were the ones that had damaged me, but the bastards that had perpetrated the rape and murder, and suddenly I had an outlet for my anger. Obvious really, but I'd somehow got that all tangled up, and then it clarified itself. That was important.

'Seeing Oliver affected by his own memory of the woman hanging from the tree, that was important, but there was something else about that, a feeling I hadn't experienced before, and I can't describe it. It was like a calmness, a stillness, I felt expanded, like I was bigger than my body, felt like I could have encompassed the world, all the people, everywhere, who are in pain. I must say something about that to Oliver. I'm not sure why I didn't at the time.

'Just thinking about it makes me feel different even now – calmer, stiller, somehow more at peace. Mmm.

'In a way it is hard to think of something else as standing out after that, and yet I know that the way Oliver listened and did not judge me when I talked about the incident in the Gulf, and as I say this I feel that peacefulness fading, was so important. I don't imagine I ever will tell anyone else, but at least another soul knows. I still wonder about his family. I still feel tearful thinking about it. I know other things happened in the heat of battle and, well, not everyone reacted as I did, or reacts as I do now as I think back.

'And, of course, that period when I was talking about Geordie. I think if he hadn't kept a strong expression, and held eye contact, I'd have ended at that session. Something about how he held my expression said something, even though I knew he probably had no idea what I would talk about. But he looked like he was trying, really trying. It suddenly felt like, yeah, maybe this guy can get real with me on this, maybe I can tell him more.

'I feel I have a long way to go. I want to make full use of the next few sessions and then, who knows. Maybe I will carry on with counselling though it wouldn't seem right with someone else. I don't know. We'll have to see. For the moment I am grateful to have met Oliver, and at a time in my life when I needed to meet him. I'm going to investigate counselling a little more, but first I have to get myself back to work, back into family life and then we'll see what the future holds.'

Afterword

When asked by Richard if I would write an Afterword to this excellent new book on counselling victims of warfare, my immediate reaction was to say that 34 years service in the Royal Navy was hardly the sort of experience suitable for such a responsible task. But then later, on reflection, I realised that my response had been based on exactly the experience he was seeking because in those 34 years not once had I come across any sort of counselling, either in my training or in the subsequent progress through my career. In fact my service experience was of a total absence of any sort of guidance on the development of emotional support skills when dealing with colleagues and subordinates in stressful situations, or importantly how one should deal with one's own inward needs for emotional support.

Until I retired in 1995, and possibly even now, the three armed forces relied heavily on a type of 'mentoring' in which leaders at each level have full responsibility for those in their charge. This mentoring, if I may call it that, is based upon the leader having both 'carrot and stick' in managing the wellbeing of his or her group. In the Royal Navy it is the Divisional System, in the Army, the Section or Platoon, and in the RAF, the Squadron organisation. For leaders the 'stick' is of course service discipline, whilst the 'carrot' is responsibility for allocating tasks and rewards, such as giving time off for sport and leisure. But the mentoring also includes monitoring the personal lives of subordinates outside the service, in particular their relationships with close family members. The service does not want distractions for the task in hand.

How does this work in practice? At 25 years old, as a young Lieutenant at sea in an aircraft carrier in the Pacific, I was woken up late one night by a 40-year-old Chief Petty Officer in great physical and mental distress, for whom I had direct divisional responsibility, asking me to deal with his news that his wife had contracted venereal disease after an affair with a next door neighbour. There and then I had to support him and reassure him so that he was able to rejoin his colleagues and get back to his job, plus a promise that I would activate the family welfare service and, if necessary, organise for him to be returned to the UK to resolve the matter. Whilst I had been given training for the last two tasks, dealing with an older, married subordinate with family problems and his considerable stress left me inwardly 'all at sea'.

My generation of servicemen would not have experienced, indeed would not have known about, counselling. For Graham in Part 2 of this book, his first meeting with Oliver is, using a military term, 'a night encounter'. He knows someone is there, but because it is dark, if not pitch black, is he friend or foe, and what are his intentions? Richard describes this encounter admirably, sensitive to the difficulty someone like Graham may have early on in establishing trust with a mental health professional.

From personal naval experience, and I am sure this applies to both the Army and Royal Air Force, feelings in stressful service situations are always suppressed and kept under firm control. During a number of dangerous situations I was conscious of my group watching my reactions as events unfolded. I was convinced that if I showed the slightest fear or doubt this would quickly transfer to my team and that the vital instinct to fight for survival would be lost. I was trained, we all were trained, to keep our feelings to ourselves.

So as the relationship between Oliver and Graham develops, the point at which Graham for the first time cries may possibly be the first time he has ever allowed his emotions to show, even possibly to his wife. He is not likely to have cried while still serving. He would probably have felt that showing such emotion would have singled him out as different, if not weak, amongst his colleagues. To this day I still recall the TV news report of the Paras burying their fallen comrades after the battle for Goose Green during the Falklands Campaign. Not a single soldier cried.

I think Richard has captured these two significant aspects in using the complex relationship between Oliver and Graham as a case study for counselling victims of warfare. It is real and compelling. For me I felt I knew where Graham had been and now, having read this excellent book, I think I know where, with expert help, he will with luck be going.

John Castle
Captain, Royal Navy (1958–95)
Barton-on-the-Heath, Gloucestershire
June 2005

Author's epilogue

This was not a book that I looked forward to writing but one that I felt had to be written. At that time I did not know how either of the counselling scenarios would develop. In fact, I wrote Part 2 first, I wanted to in a sense use it to get into the theme, although, of course, Part 1 took its own direction and evolved in its own way. I actually wrote the book quite quickly as well. It has been important to stay in touch with the characters, to not lose the threads, so to speak, the streams of consciousness that link the various experiences being described. It therefore became an intense process. Yet a deeply satisfying one as it extends and expands my own understanding and practice as I learn through research and through the responses that emerge from the counsellors and from their supervisors.

There are so many people in our world, like Ania and Graham, each seeking to live with experiences that have deeply and profoundly affected them. There are so many victims of war, people deeply affected by the horrendous events that they have experienced and which the human psyche does its best to contain and to survive, sometimes by trying to keep that experience out of awareness. At other times the experience gets stuck, so intense that it is imprinted on the person in such a way that its presence does not diminish, but remains dominant and forming a 'configuration within self' with its own associated constellation of thoughts, feelings and behaviours.

Is it right to describe the military man as a 'victim' of war? I am sure that some will disagree, perhaps many. I'm unsure what is the best language to use. War is messy. It can draw out strength and courage as much as it can provide a vehicle for brutality and sadistic tendencies to be expressed. Maybe it is our humanity that is at risk of becoming the real victim? Or can there be growth in spite of, or even as a result of, war experiences? I am sure both can be true.

I want to say something about discipline, which I have mentioned previously in the text. Military forces need to be disciplined, and the individual in a combat situation needs self-discipline. And it is strange to think in the same paragraph of the self-discipline needed to be an effective person-centred therapist. In no way do I wish to compare the two types of discipline. It is simply very important for counsellors working with people from a military background and with combat experience to have in mind that they are working with people whose self-discipline may be such that it forms a formidable barrier to the sharing and expressing of emotion and this may present difficulties.

As with all the books in the *Living Therapy* series, *Counselling Victims of Warfare: person-centred dialogues* has profoundly affected me. I have had to engage with the characters in a way that has been upsetting, but I am grateful for this for it has ensured that they have felt real and substantial as persons, albeit fictitious. And, as always, at the end of a book they are so alive that I am left wondering what their future will hold. Well, there are many Anias and Grahams in the world, seeking a way to come to terms with the past that has so invaded their present, and seeking a way forward into a future that will be fulfilling and where they may feel some relief from the horrors of their past.

And there are many Marias, children who are the product of acts of atrocity, many of whom are in orphanages, or struggling to survive as best they can on the streets in different parts of the world wherever warfare has occurred, or fighting with militias themselves, having been trained to kill from an early age.

I do not have an answer to warfare, but it is so much a part of the individual and collective human experience. Many years ago I read a passage that, I think, sums up what is needed, and maybe one day we will see it happen: 'I ask you to drop your antagonisms and your antipathies, your hatreds and your racial differences, and attempt to think in terms of the one family, the one life, and the one humanity' (Bailey, 1936, p. 188). Until enough people respond positively to that call we will have wars, and victims of warfare. The flow of hatred, the desire for revenge and retribution, the atmospheres of distrust, will continue to provide the climate in which violent confrontation can emerge.

Later in his life Rogers undertook a lot of work with groups to resolve conflict, applying the principles of the person-centred approach. His pioneering work made a difference to people's lives, providing an opportunity for people to hear and understand each other's pain and, as a result, discover their own compassion for those who stood 'on the other side'. He established methods of working to help people to build community based on person-centred principles. He was actually nominated for a Nobel Peace Prize. Centres such as that represented in Part 1 are excellent places to provide reconciliation groups along the lines pioneered by Rogers.

The world needs people to work with the victims of warfare either one-to-one or through groups. I hope that this book has helped to prepare the reader, or enhance the reader's ability, to work in this area of human experience.

References

Agni Yoga Society (1959) *Aum* (2e). Agni Yoga Society Inc., New York.

Ahrenfeld RH (1958) *Psychiatry in the British Army in the Second World War*. Routledge & Kegan Paul, London.

Bailey AA (1936) *A Treatise on the Seven Rays*. Volume 1: *Esoteric Psychology I*. Lucis Press Ltd, London.

Bailey AA (1960) *A Treatise on the Seven Rays*. Volume 5: *The Rays and the Initiations*. Lucis Press Ltd, London.

Barrett-Lennard GT (1998) *Carl Rogers Helping System: journey & substance*. Sage, London.

Bentall R (ed.) (1990) The syndromes and symptons of psychosis. In: *Reconstructing Schizophrenia*. Routledge, London.

Binneveld H (1997) *From Shellshock to Combat Stress: a comparative history of military psychiatry*. Amsterdam University Press, Amsterdam.

Bozarth J (1998) *Person-Centred Therapy: a revolutionary paradigm*. PCCS Books, Ross-on-Wye.

Bozarth J (2002) Empirically supported treatments: epitome of the specificity myth. In: JC Watson, RN Goldman and MS Warner (eds). *Client-centred and Experiential Psychotherapy in the 21st Century: advances in theory, research and practice*. PCCS Books, Ross-on-Wye, pp. 68–181.

Bozarth J and Wilkins P (eds) (2001) *Rogers' Therapeutic Conditions: evolution, theory and practice*. Volume 3: *Congruence*. PCCS Books, Ross-on-Wye.

Bracken P and Petty C (1998) *Rethinking the Trauma of War*. Free Association Books, London.

Bryant-Jefferies R (2001) *Counselling the Person Beyond the Alcohol Problem*. Jessica Kingsley Publishers, London.

Bryant-Jefferies R (2003a) *Counselling a Survivor of Child Sexual Abuse: a person-centred dialogue*. Radcliffe Medical Press, Oxford.

Bryant-Jefferies R (2003b) *Time Limited Therapy in Primary Care: a person-centred dialogue*. Radcliffe Medical Press, Oxford.

Bryant-Jefferies R (2003c) *Problem Drinking: a person-centred dialogue*. Radcliffe Medical Press, Oxford.

Bryant-Jefferies R (2005a) *Personal and Professional: person-centred counselling supervision*. Radcliffe Publishing, Oxford.

Bryant-Jefferies R (2005b) *Responding to a Serious Mental Health Problem: person-centred dialogues.* Radcliffe Publishing, Oxford.

Bryant-Jefferies R (2005c) *Workplace Counselling in the NHS: person-centred dialogues.* Radcliffe Publishing, Oxford.

Culpin M (1920) *Psychoneuroses of War and Peace.* Cambridge University Press, Cambridge.

Embleton Tudor L, Keemar K, Tudor K *et al.* (2004) *The Person-Centred Approach: a contemporary introduction.* Palgrave MacMillan, Basingstoke.

Emerson RW (1987) *Social Aims: works of Ralph Waldo Emerson.* Routledge and Sons Ltd, London.

Evans R (1975) *Carl Rogers: the man and his ideas.* Dutton and Co., New York.

Gaylin N (2001) *Family, Self and Psychotherapy: a person-centred perspective.* PCCS Books, Ross-on-Wye.

Haugh S and Merry T (eds) (2001) *Rogers' Therapeutic Conditions: evolution, theory and practice.* Volume 2: *Empathy.* PCCS Books, Ross-on-Wye.

Hallett R (1990) Melancholia and Depression: a brief history and analysis of contemporary confusions. Unpublished Masters Thesis, University of East London.

Hallam RS (1983) Agoraphobia: deconstructing a clinical syndrome. *Bulletin of the British Psychological Society.* **36**: 337–40.

Hallam RS (1989) Classification and research into panic. In: R Baker and M McFadyen (eds) *Panic Disorder.* Wiley, Chichester.

Hollis M (2004) Personal communication.

Janoff-Bulman R (1992) *Shattered Assumptions: toward new psychology of trauma.* The Free Press, New York.

Joseph S (2003) A person-centred approach to post-traumatic stress. *Person-Centred Practice.* **11**(2): 70–5.

Kirschenbaum H (2005) The current status of Carl Rogers and the person-centred approach. *Psychotherapy.* **42**(1): 37–51.

Kirschenbaum H and Henderson VL (1990) *The Carl Rogers Reader.* Constable, London.

Kutchins H and Kirk S (1997) *Making us Crazy: DSM: the psychiatric bible and the creation of mental disorders.* The Free Press/Simon Schuster, New York.

Linley PA and Joseph S (2002) Post-traumatic growth. *Counselling and Psychotherapy Journal.* **13**(1): 14–17.

Mearns D (1999) Person centred therapy with configurations of self. *Counselling.* **10**: 147–8.

Mearns D and Thorne B (1988) *Person-Centred Counselling in Action.* Sage, London.

Mearns D and Thorne B (1999) *Person-Centred Counselling in Action* (2e). Sage, London.

Mearns D and Thorne B (2000) *Person-Centred Therapy Today.* Sage, London.

Merry T (2001) Congruence and the supervision of client-centred therapists. In: G Wyatt (ed.) *Rogers' Therapeutic Conditions: evolution, theory and practice.* Volume 1: *Congruence.* PCCS Books, Ross-on-Wye, pp. 174–83.

Merry T (2002) *Learning and Being in Person-Centred Counselling* (2e). PCCS Books, Ross-on-Wye.

Myers CS (1940) *Shell Shock in France 1914–1918*. Cambridge University Press, Cambridge.

Palmer IP (2002) Psychotherapy, the psychology of trauma and army psychiatry since 1904. In: C Feltham (ed.) *What's the Good of Counselling and Psychotherapy?* Sage, London, pp. 225–39.

Patterson (2000) *Understanding Psychotherapy: fifty years of client-centred theory and practice.* PCCS Books, Ross-on-Wye.

Purton C (2002) Person-centred therapy without the core conditions. *Counselling and Psychotherapy Journal.* **13**: 6–9.

Rivers WHR (1916) The repression of war experience. *Lancet.* **2**: 173–7.

Rivers WHR (1918) War neurosis and military training. *Mental Hygiene.* **2**(4): 513–33.

Rogers CR (1942) *Counselling and Psychotherapy: newer concepts in practice.* Houghton-Mifflin Co., Boston, MA.

Rogers CR (1951) *Client-Centred Therapy.* Constable, London.

Rogers CR (1957) The necessary and sufficient conditions of therapeutic personality change. *Journal Consulting Psychology.* **21**: 95–103.

Rogers CR (1959) A theory of therapy, personality and interpersonal relationships as developed in the client-centred framework. In: S Koch (ed.) *Psychology: a study of a science.* Volume 3: *Formulations of the person and the social context.* McGraw-Hill, New York, pp. 185–246.

Rogers CR (1967) *On Becoming a Person.* Constable, London. Original work 1961.

Rogers CR (1980) *A Way of Being.* Houghton-Mifflin Co., Boston, MA.

Rogers CR (1986) A client-centered/person-centered approach to therapy. In: I Kutash and A Wolfe (eds) *Psychotherapists' Casebook.* Jossey Bass, San Francisco, pp. 236–57.

Shephard B (2000) *A War of Nerves.* Jonathan Cape, London.

Slade PD and Cooper R (1979) Some difficulties with the term 'schizophrenia': an alternative model. *British Journal Social and Clinical Psychology.* **18**: 309–17.

Tudor K and Worrall M (2004) *Freedom to Practise: person-centred approaches to supervision.* PCCS Books, Ross-on-Wye.

Velleman R (2001) *Counselling for Alcohol Problems* (2e). Sage, London.

Warner M (2000) Person-centred therapy at the difficult edge: a developmentally based model of fragile and dissociated process. In: D Mearns and B Thorne (eds) *Person-Centred Therapy Today.* Sage Publications, London.

Warner M (2002) Psychological contact, meaningful process and human nature. In: G Wyatt and P Sanders (eds) *Rogers' Therapeutic Conditions: evolution, theory and practice.* Volume 4: *Contact and Perception.* PCCS Books, Ross-on-Wye, pp. 76–95.

Wiener M (1989) Psychopathology reconsidered: depression interpreted as psychosocial interactions. *Clinical Psychology Review.* **9**: 295–321.

Wilkins P (2003) *Person Centred Therapy in Focus.* Sage, London.

Wyatt G (ed.) (2001) *Rogers' Therapeutic Conditions: evolution, theory and practice*. Volume 1: *Congruence*. PCCS Books, Ross-on-Wye.

Wyatt G and Sanders P (eds) (2002) *Rogers' Therapeutic Conditions: evolution, theory and practice*. Volume 4: *Contact and Perception*. PCCS Books, Ross-on-Wye.

Further reading

- Ager A (ed.) (1999) *Refugees: perspectives on the experience of forced migration*. Cassell Academic, London.

- Arcel L and Simunkovic G (eds) (1998) *War Violence, Trauma and the Coping Process: armed conflict in Europe and survivor responses*. International Rehabilitation Council for Torture Victims, Copenhagen.

- Bracken P and Petty C (eds) (1998) *Rethinking the Trauma of War*. Free Association Books/Save the Children Fund, London.

- Langer J (ed.) (1997) *The Bend in the Road: refugees writing*. Five Leaves Publications, Nottingham.

- McCallin M (ed.) (1996) *The Psychological Well-being of Refugee Children: research, practice and policy issues* (2e). International Catholic Child Bureau, Geneva.

- McCarthy J (ed.) (1999) *Captured Voices*. Medical Foundation for the Care of Victims of Torture, London.

- Mertus J (ed.) (1997) *The Suitcase: refugee voices from Bosnia and Croatia*. University of California Press, Berkeley, California.

- Peel M (2004) *Rape as a Method of Torture*. Medical Foundation for the Care of Victims of Torture, London.

- Staehr A and Staehr M (1995) *Counselling Torture Survivors*. International Rehabilitation Council for Torture Victims, Copenhagen.

- Tolfree D (ed.) (1996) *Restoring Playfulness: different approaches to assisting children who are psychologically affected by war or displacement*. Radda Barnen, Stockholm.

- van der Veer G (1998) *Counselling and Therapy with Refugees and Victims of Trauma: psychological problems of victims of war, torture and repression*. John Wiley & Sons, Chichester.

Useful contacts

Person-centred

Association for the Development of the Person-Centered Approach (ADPCA)
Email: adpca-web@signs.portents.com
Website: www.adpca.org

An international association, with members in 27 countries, for those interested in the development of client-centred therapy and the person-centred approach.

British Association for the Person-Centred Approach (BAPCA)
Bm-BAPCA
London WC1N 3XX
Tel: 01989 770948
Email: info@bapca.org.uk
Website: www.bapca.org.uk

National association promoting the person-centred approach. Publishes the journal *Person-centred Practice* and a regular newsletter *Person-to-Person*.

World Association for Person-Centered and Experiential Psychotherapy and Counselling
Email: secretariat@pce-world.org
Website: www.pce-world.org

The Association aims to provide a worldwide forum for those professionals in science and practice who are committed to, and embody in their work, the theoretical principles of the person-centred approach first postulated by Carl Rogers. The Association publishes *Person-centred and Experiential Psychotherapies*, an international journal which 'creates a dialogue among different parts of the person-centred/experiential therapy tradition, supporting, informing and challenging academics and practitioners with the aim of the development of these approaches in a broad professional, scientific and political context'.

Person Centred Therapy Scotland
Tel: 0870 7650871
Email: info@pctscotland.co.uk
Website: www.pctscotland.co.uk

An association of person-centred therapists in Scotland which offers training and networking opportunities to members, with the aim of fostering high standards of professional practice.

Victims of warfare

Combat Stress
Tyrwhitt House
Oaklawn Road
Leatherhead
Surrey KT22 0BX
Tel: 01372 841600
Email: contactus@combatstress.org.uk
Website: www.combatstress.com

The Ex-Services Mental Welfare Society, Combat Stress, exists to serve the psychiatric casualties of military service. For over 80 years it has been the only services charity specialising in helping those of all ranks from the Armed Forces and the Merchant Navy suffering from psychological disability as a result of their service. It works through a national network of welfare officers, visiting clients at home in order to establish how best they can improve their quality of life, and through three treatment centres, providing rehabilitative treatment which aims to help the victim cope with his or her disabilities and to enjoy a better quality of life.

Joint Council for the Welfare of Immigrants
115 Old Street
London EC1V 9RT
Tel: 020 7251 8708
Fax: 020 7251 8707
Email: info@jcwi.org.uk
Website: www.jcwi.org.uk

The Joint Council for the Welfare of Immigrants is an independent national voluntary organisation, campaigning for justice and combating racism in immigration and asylum law and policy. It provides free advice and casework, training courses and a range of publications.

NHS Services
Many parts of the country now offer specific refugee support and counselling services. For information on what is available in your area, contact your GP or local Primary Care Trust.

Refugee Council
Head Office & One Stop Service:
240–250 Ferndale Road
London SW9 8BB
Tel: 020 7346 6700
Fax: 020 7346 6778
Email: info@refugeecouncil.org.uk
Website: www.refugeecouncil.org.uk

Yorkshire & Humberside region office:
Ground Floor
Hurley House
1 Dewsbury Road
Leeds LS11 5DQ
Tel: 0113 244 9404
Fax: 0113 246 5229

Eastern region office:
First floor
4–8 Museum Street
Ipswich IP1 1HT
Tel: 01473 297900
Fax: 01473 217334

West Midlands region office:
First Floor
Smithfield House
Digbeth
Birmingham B5 6BS
Tel: 0121 622 1515
Fax: 0121 622 4061

Advice line: Open Monday, Tuesday, Thursday, Friday, 10 am–1 pm and 2–4 pm, Wednesday 2–4 pm. Tel: 020 7346 6777.

The One Stop Service advice line is operated by advisers with experience in asylum and immigration matters. It aims to provide advice and information on a wide range of issues, including social security, family reunion, identity and travel documentation, education, housing, legal issues and information about refugee community organisations. The advice line welcomes calls from both individuals and organisations.

For legal reasons it cannot offer advice via its advice line, but should be able to refer you to someone who can.

The Medical Foundation for the Care of Victims of Torture
111 Isledon Road
Islington
London N7 7JW

Tel: 020 7697 7777
Fax: 020 7697 7799
Website: www.torturecare.org.uk

Medical Foundation Northwest
The Angel
St Philips Place
Chapel Street
Salford M3 6FA
Tel: 0161 839 8090
Fax: 0161 839 7020

Founded in 1985, the Medical Foundation for the Care of Victims of Torture provides care and rehabilitation to survivors of torture and other forms of organised violence. It aims to:

- provide survivors of torture in the UK with medical treatment, practical assistance and psychotherapeutic support
- document evidence of torture
- provide training for health professionals working with torture survivors
- educate the public and decision-makers about torture and its consequences
- ensure that Britain honours its international obligations towards survivors of torture, asylum seekers and refugees.

Index